Saoussen Chouchene
Mezrigui Rihem
Maroua Chaouch

Chediak-Higashi syndrome: From genetics to treatment

Saoussen Chouchene
Mezrigui Rihem
Maroua Chaouch

Chediak-Higashi syndrome: From genetics to treatment

Comprehensive Analcysis and Therapeutic Challenges

ScienciaScripts

Imprint

Cover image: www.ingimage.com

This book is a translation from the original published under ISBN 978-620-6-72273-1.

Publisher:
Sciencia Scripts
is a trademark of
Dodo Books Indian Ocean Ltd. and OmniScriptum S.R.L publishing group

120 High Road, East Finchley, London, N2 9ED, United Kingdom
Str. Armeneasca 28/1, office 1, Chisinau MD-2012, Republic of Moldova, Europe
Printed at: see last page
ISBN: 978-620-8-13989-6

CONTENTS

INTRODUCTION

Chediak-Higashi syndrome (CHS) is a primary immune deficiency characterised by oculocutaneous albinism, recurrent infections, a tendency to haemorrhage and progressive neurological abnormalities. It is a rare autosomal recessive disorder of lysosomal trafficking linked to mutations in the LYST (lysosomal trafficking regulator) gene located on the long arm of chromosome 1 and coding for the LYST protein involved in the synthesis, transport and fusion of cytoplasmic vesicles **[1-5]**.

The first case of this syndrome was reported in 1943, followed by around 500 cases worldwide. 85% to 90% of patients had the classic form characterised by the development, from the first decade of life, of a macrophagic syndrome or haemophagocytic lymphohistiocytosis (HHL) heralding the accelerated phase of the disease. On the other hand, 10-15% develop the attenuated form, dominated mainly by neurological manifestations **[6-8]**.

The pathognomonic sign of this syndrome is the presence of bulky intra-cytoplasmic blue-grey or pinkish-grey inclusions in the cytoplasm of leukocytes, melanocytes and platelets **[9,10]**.

Furthermore, the vital prognosis of the disease is very severe, and current management of CHS is limited to symptomatic means. However, allogeneic haematopoietic stem cell transplantation (HSCT) allows survival beyond 20 years by reducing the risk of macrophagic activation syndrome **[1]**.

1. HISTORY

CHS was first described in 1943 by Antonio Beguez César, a Cuban paediatrician, who studied the cases of three siblings who bore the main clinical features of this syndrome and presented with atypical enlarged granules in the leukocytes. In 1948, other cases were described by Steinbrinck, a Cuban haematologist **[11-13]**.

A few years later, Moises Chediak (a French doctor) and Ototaka Higashi (a Japanese physiotherapist) described cases characterised by a poor distribution of myeloperoxidase in neutrophil granules and specified the haematological characteristics of the disease, which prompted Sato to associate their names with the anomaly **[14-18]**.

Four out of thirteen children were affected in the family studied by Chediak and three out of six in the family described by Higashi. These affected children presented with partial albinism, photophobia associated with nystagmus and an increased red reflex of the eyes following exposure to light. They were unusually susceptible to pyogenic infections, with reports of death before the age of seven following the development of hepatosplenomegaly **[16,17,19]**.

In 1964, Kritzler et al **[20]** characterised the "accelerated phase" of the disease by the presence of haemophagocytic lymphohistiocytosis, observed in around 85% of cases.

In 1967, Lutzner et al **[21]** first recognised the beige mouse as an animal model of CHS, characterised by a pigmentary anomaly in the coat, reduced ocular acuity and the presence of giant lysosomes, the distribution of which was subsequently studied by Oliver and Essner **[22]**.

In 1968, Sung et al. reported neurological manifestations in four CHS patients.

In 1976, Buchanan et al. studied platelet function defects in CHS patients for the first time **[23]**.

In 1983, Griscelli and Virelizier performed a bone marrow transplant in a three-year-old child **[24]**.

Prenatal diagnosis was made in 1992 by Diukman et al, who measured lysosomes positive for acid phosphatase in amniocytes and chorionic villi and found that lysosomes were significantly larger in CHS. Then, in 1993, Durandy et al. examined fetal scalp biopsies and fetal blood samples by light and electron microscopy **[23]**.

The first treatment protocol for LHH was introduced in 1994, and over the last few decades a growing understanding of the underlying biological mechanisms of LHH has led to the standardisation of treatment and management protocols, resulting in improved survival **[25]**.

In 1995, Haddad et al. summarised the results of allogeneic bone marrow transplantation in ten children with CHS. Transplantation was successful in seven children, six of whom received HLA-identical marrow **[23]**.

However, the genetic defect responsible for this syndrome was only identified and mapped on the human chromosome in 1996 **[6]**.

To date, 74 mutations in the CHS1 gene have been described, including nonsense mutations, deletions, insertions and splice sites **[12]**.

2. EPIDEMIOLOGY

CHS is a rare disease, with fewer than 600 cases reported worldwide **[25-27].** In the United States, fewer than 30 patients have been described **[23]**. Similarly, in China, around 50 cases have been reported in recent decades **[6]**.

In Japan, a total of fifteen patients with CHS were diagnosed between 2000 and 2010, and the data from these patients was collected and analysed, leading to the conclusion that one or two patients with CHS will be newly diagnosed each year **[28,29].**

However, the exact prevalence of CHS remains difficult to determine, as some cases have been reported more than once in the literature. Furthermore, the phenotypic variability that has been observed more recently suggests that many affected individuals may be unreported **[15,30]**.

The syndrome affects both sexes and all breeds **[11,15,31]**. Similarly, all age groups may be affected. However, it should be noted that the classic form of this disease mainly affects children, with an average age of onset of around six years, and most of these patients die before the age of ten; 50% of these cases involve children from consanguineous marriages **[11,15,32]**.

3. CLASSIFICATION

CHS is classified into two forms: the classic or infantile form and the atypical or adult form **[6,7,33]**.

3.1. Shape classic

The classic form accounts for around 85% of cases. It is characterised by the frequency of severe infections, the presence of albinism, bleeding and haemophagocytic lymphohistiocytosis (HHL), also known as the accelerated phase, which is characterised by fever, hepatosplenomegaly, bi- or pancytopenia and haemophagocytosis. HHL appears at an early age and generally leads to death within the first decade of life **[33,34]**. Hence the poor prognosis of this classic form unless a bone marrow transplant is performed **[11]**.

3.2. Form atypical

The atypical or adult form has been estimated to account for 15% of all CHS patients, but may be under-diagnosed **[6]**.

Patients with this form have a less severe clinical course. They have a lower frequency of infections in childhood, subtle alterations in pigmentation and survive into adulthood without experiencing the accelerated phase. Nevertheless, during adolescence or adulthood, they develop progressive, inconstant and non-specific neurological symptoms **[6,35]**.

Like the clinical manifestations, the cellular manifestations may be attenuated in patients with the atypical form **[35]**.

4. PATHOPHYSIOLOGY

4.1. Reminder physiology

4.1.1. The endolysosomal system

The endolysosomal system plays an important role in metabolic control, macromolecule degradation and signalling. Several types of cell adapt their system endolysosomal system their conferring This is the case for melanosomes in pigment cells, granules in platelets, Weibel-Palade endothelial bodies (WPBs) and lytic granules in cytotoxic cells, particularly cytotoxic T lymphocytes (CTLs) **[36]**. Lysosome-related organelles (LROs) are characterised by diversity not only in morphology and content, but also in the origin of their membranes and the mechanisms required for their formation, maturation and secretion. For example, some LROs appear to derive mainly from endosomes (e.g. melanosomes), while others originate from the secretory pathway while acquiring from contents additional content from the system endolysosomal system (e.g. WPBs and neuronal dense nuclear granules). In addition, lysosomes are essential components of various cell types, including melanocytes, platelets, granulocytes, cTLs and NK cells. They help secrete specific proteins and peptides, depending on the cell type **[37]**.

4.1.2. The traffic regulatory protein lysosomal

The LYST (Lysosomal trafficking regulator) protein, also known as CHS1, is a cytoplasmic protein that influences the biogenesis of the endosomal compartment, affecting the terminal maturation of secretory lysosomes. It is expressed in all human cells, with higher levels in bone marrow, cerebellum, spleen and thymus. The protein is composed of 3801 amino acids and has a molecular weight of 430 kDa. The N-terminus of the LYST protein contains a series of Armadillo (ARM) and Huntingtin (HEAT) helix repeats. These repeats are important for mediating membrane associations and vesicle transport. The

C-terminus of the protein contains three domains: a pleckstrin homologous domain (PH), a Beige and Chediak-Higashi domain (BEACH) which contains a 'WIDL' consensus amino acid segment (W:tryptophan, I:isoleucine D:aspartic acid, L: leucine) as well as several other conserved amino acids that define members of the BEACH protein family and a region of seven WD-40 (tryptophan-aspartic acid) repeat motifs indicative of a protein-protein interaction domain (**Figure 1**). Studies on proteins with BEACH domains have revealed part of the functional role of these domains and suggest their primary involvement in vesicular trafficking. [**1,23,38-40**] .

Although the molecular understanding and exact biological role of the LYST protein is still very limited, the combined PH-BEACH motifs are thought to be involved in different aspects of vesicular trafficking and, therefore, probably play a crucial role in the regulation of lysosomal size, in membrane fusion and fission events as a scaffolding protein and in vesicular secretion. Previous studies have also suggested that LYST is required for sorting resident endosomal proteins in late multivesicular endosomes **[41-43]**.

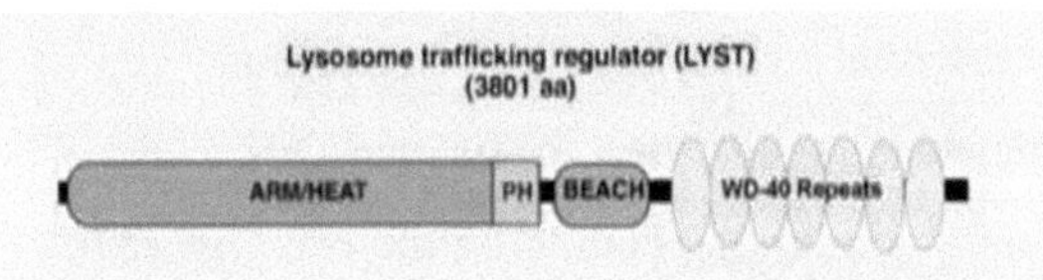

Figure1Domainsofraficlysosomalregulatory protein and Chediak Higashi 1 syndrome [1].

ARM: Armadillo; HEAT: Huntingtin; PH: homologous pleckstrin; BEACH: Beige and Chediak- Higashi; WD-40: tryptophan-aspartic acid; LYST: lysosomal trafficking regulator

4.2. Pathogenesis

4.2.1. Pathophysiological mechanism of Chediak-Higashi syndrome

In the CHS, mutation of the gene encoding the LYST protein disrupts the synthesis of lysosomal traffic proteins and affects the size and function of lysosomes, promoting aberrant vesicle fusion and defective transport of lysosomes to the site of action in a wide range of cells, such as immune system cells, melanocytes, neurons and platelets **[11,15,27,32,44,45]**. These defects then result in enlarged, non-functional lysosomes and abnormal lysosome-related organelles including platelet and neutrophil granules, melanocyte melanosomes, major histocompatibility complex (MHC) class II compartments and also the lysosomes of other leukocytes and fibroblasts, and this is the main cellular feature of CHS **[15,30]**.

Two different models are presented to explain the dysregulation of lysosome size. A first model suggests that LYST is required for appropriate fusion events. This model is supported by studies in human cells which reveal that the interaction of LYST with proteins involved in attachment, docking and fusion mechanisms is impaired in the CHS. The other model suggests that LYST may contribute to lysosomal membrane fission events instead of fusion. This hypothesis was supported for the first time by studies of LYST overexpression in mice, which causes fragmentation and peripheral dispersion of lysosomes, leading to a reduction in lysosome size. These observations led the authors to conclude that the rate of lysosomal fission is positively regulated by LYST. Depletion of LYST in human HeLa and U2OS cell lines leads to fewer and larger lysosomes, supporting the idea that the lysosomes observed in CHS patient cells are caused by loss-of-function mutations in LYST. Interestingly, depletion of LYST in in human cells has no effect on the fusion of lysosomes with endosomes and autophagosomes, on their degradation capacity or on trafficking via autophagy, endocytosis or retrograde transport. Another cellular defect observed in fibroblasts from CHS patients and beige mice is a deficiency in plasma membrane resealing after injury. Plasma membrane injury is repaired by a Ca2+-dependent exocytosis mechanism, involving an increase in intracellular Ca2+ that triggers the fusion of small peripheral lysosomes with the plasma membrane. This suggests that lysosome enlargement may deplete the small peripheral lysosomes that are preferentially involved in Ca2+-triggered exocytosis in fibroblasts **[1,26,41,46]**.

The underlying biochemical abnormality has not been determined, but studies suggest that abnormal regulation or proteolysis of protein kinase C (PKC) by increased ceramide production is responsible for the formation of giant granules, leading to abnormal cellular phenotypes responsible for the beige phenotype **[26]**.

At the cellular level, LYST interacts with certain cytoplasmic proteins that play important roles in the regulation of vesicular transport or signal transduction, such as the substrate for tyrosine kinase regulated by hepatocyte growth factor (HRS), casein kinase II (CK2), calmodulin (CALM) and 14-3-3 proteins. HRS inhibits exocytosis by binding to SNAP25, a component of the SNARE protein complex that plays an important role in vesicle docking and fusion. In the normal cell, LYST forms a complex with HRS, and the HRS-LYST complex is unable to bind SNAP25. CALM plays an important role in membrane fusion. In addition, mediation of HRS activity by LYST and CALM complexes is thought to enhance SNAP25-regulated membrane docking and fusion **(Figure 2).** In the SCH, the absence of LYST could prevent the juxtaposition of HRS and CALM, potentiating the inhibition of SNAP25 by HRS, and thus inhibiting membrane docking and fusion **[47]**.

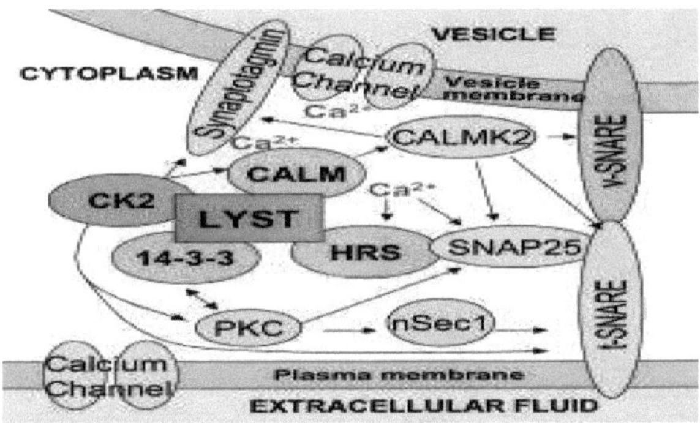

Figure2:Interactions of the lysosomal traffic regulatory protein with proteins that regulate vesicle docking and fusion in exocytosis [48].
CALM: Calmodulin; LYST: Lysosomal trafficking regulator; CK2: CaseinKinase2; NSec1: N- Selenocysteine1; CALMK2: Calmodulin Kinase 2; t-SNARE: target-soluble N-ethylmaleimide- sensitive factor attachment protein receptors; v-SNARE: vesicular-soluble N-ethylmaleimide-sensitive factor attachment protein receptors; SNAP25: synaptosome-associated protein of 25 kD; HRS: Hepatocyte growth factor Regulated tyrosine kinase Substrate;

A previous study identified 21 proteins that interact with LYST using a yeast two-hybrid screen. The R1104X mutation in LYST results in a loss of interaction with 18 proteins, which probably play a key role in vesicular attachment, margination, fusion, phosphorylation and signal transduction. The LYST N2535KfsX2 truncation results in the loss of nine interacting proteins involved in neurodegenerative disorders, transcription regulation and signal transduction **[48]**.

4.2.2. Pathogenesis of albinism

Pigmentation of the eye, skin and hair is the result of melanin pigment production in melanocytes. Melanin-producing cells contain specialised lysosome-like organelles called melanosomes, which deposit the melanin pigment in a mature state **[49]**. Once in the keratinocytes, melanosomes are distributed and, in response to UV rays, strategically positioned on the "sun-exposed" side of the nuclei to form umbrella-like structures **[50,51]**.

Melanosome formation, maturation and trafficking are crucial for pigmentation. Defects in melanosome trafficking can lead to depigmentation syndromes such as Chediak-Higashi syndrome (CHS). In the epidermal melanocytes of people with CHS, the enlarged melanosomes accumulate in the perinuclear zone of the melanocytes and are not transferred to the surrounding keratinocytes, which could explain the cutaneous hypopigmentation observed in this syndrome. In some patients, patchy skin hypopigmentation or mottled hyperpigmentation may be observed **[1,6,30]**.

4.2.3. Pathogenesis of immunodeficiency and recurrent infections CHS is well recognised as a primary immune deficiency (PID) with pathognomonic giant inclusions in leukocytes **[1,52]**. Patients with CHS have normal or reduced numbers of NK cells with reduced function, a defect in LTc function, in addition to neutropenia and defective neutrophil function **[25,53]**.

The giant granules present in the neutrophils of CHS patients do not properly release their contents following bacterial or viral infection **[1,54,55]**.

In addition, poor mobilisation from bone marrow, reduced deformability leading to defective chemotaxis, and delayed phagolysosomal fusion, result in reduced bactericidal activity **[25]**.

In addition, the presence of enlarged lysosomes and abnormal organelles impairs the cytotoxic activity of T lymphocytes and NK cells, leading to the development of potentially fatal HHH **[1]**.

Lymphocytes containing these large granules function poorly in antibody-dependent cell-mediated cytolysis **[15]**.

Analysis of cytotoxic T lymphocytes has suggested that the early stages of granule formation are normal. The defect in enlarged granules associated with CHS is seen at maturity, in the secretory granules **[56]**.

Lymphocyte cytotoxicity is a highly regulated process, requiring the formation of an immunological synapse (IS) between the lymphocyte and the target cell, followed by reorganisation of the lymphocyte cytoskeleton to move the microtubule organisation centre to the IS. This ensures microtubule-assisted directional transport of specialised secretory lysosomes (lytic granules) containing soluble cytolytic proteins and their exocytosis to the IS, which promotes destruction of the target cell. In CHS patients, the cytotoxic granules of LTc have limited mobility and fail to degranulate in the IS. In addition, peptide loading onto MHC class II molecules and antigen presentation are delayed **[30]**.

The secretory capacity of cytotoxic granules was restored by increasing the expression of effectors of the exocytosis machinery, suggesting that LYST may regulate the trafficking of effectors required for the terminal maturation of lytic granules containing perforins into secretory granules suitable for exocytosis **[1]**. With regard to NK cells, elimination of LYST in a human line of these cells resulted in enlargement of the lytic granules, alteration of the integrity of the endolysosomal compartments, defective exocytosis and inhibition of the cytotoxicity of these cells. In NK cells, it has been shown that in the classic presentation, the granules are fewer in number but extremely large in size. However, in atypical cases, the granules may be more numerous and smaller, but still more prominent than normal **[33]**.

These results could explain why LYST function is required for lysosomal biogenesis but not required during the early activation phase of cytotoxic cells leading to the formation of an IS to kill the target cell. These data also suggest that an enlarged lytic granule may present a physical barrier to degranulation at the IS leading to impaired cytotoxicity **[1]**.

An analysis of 21 CHS patients showed a similar degree of impairment of granule exocytosis in LTc and NK cells, despite differences in the number and size of granules in these two cell types. However, cytotoxic function was more severely affected in NK cells than in LTc cells. It should be noted that the cytotoxic function of NK cells is significantly impaired in patients with HCL, but that there are variations in the development of HCL, which are probably due to differences in the cytotoxic capacity of LTc cells **[1]**.

Mutations in the LYST gene may also contribute to defective TLR signalling and a defective immune-inflammatory response, leading to frequent and severe infections. The dysregulated immune-inflammatory response in gingival fibroblasts may have partially contributed to the periodontitis observed in CHS patients **[57]**. Apart from neutrophils, fibroblasts, one of the most abundant resident cells in periodontal tissues, form the first line of defence against micro-organisms. In addition to their structural role in synthesising and remodelling the extracellular matrix, fibroblasts secrete and respond to cytokines, chemokines and growth factors. Although several studies have focused on the effects of LYST mutations on immune cells, the effects on fibroblasts remain unclear. Previous studies have associated altered NK cell cytotoxicity with the pathogenesis of periodontitis in several genetic diseases **[57]**.

4.2.4. Pathogenesis of haemorrhages

Outside the accelerated phase, platelet counts are generally within the normal range. However, platelet function is impaired, resulting in prolonged bleeding time due to platelet dense granule deficiency, with enlarged, irregularly shaped dense bodies in some platelets. Thrombocytopenia may also occur as a result of platelet haemophagocytosis, increasing the risk of haemorrhage **[15,26,30]**.

4.2.5. Pathogenesis of neurological disorders

The mechanisms of the neurological manifestations of CHS are not always clear. It has been suggested that these manifestations result directly from defective LYST protein in neurons and glial cells, or from infiltration of lymphocyte tissue during the accelerated phase of the disease. Indeed, the defect in lysosomal exocytosis and membrane repair leads to cytoplasmic inclusions resembling giant lysosomes in neurons and the progressive accumulation of toxic substances leading to oxidative damage and neuronal cell death **[7]**. In addition, the aberrant accumulation of lysosomes interferes with membrane trafficking, which is essential for neuronal viability and axonal transport mechanisms. At autopsy, adults with CHS showed neuronal degeneration involving the olivary nuclei and cerebellar cortex. Murine models of homozygous missense mutations in the LYST gene showed predominant neurological phenotypes, including lower motor performance scores than controls, with accumulation of giant lysosomes in neuronal cells and intracytoplasmic inclusions in Purkinje cells of the cerebellum and motor cortex **[58]**. Another study revealed that the LYST genotype significantly influenced the number of Purkinje cells. Purkinje cell deficiency was detected mainly in the anterior lobules compared with those of the posterior cerebellum **[59]**.

Autopsy studies of four children with the classic form of CHS showed granules of lysosomes and lipofuscin in spinal ganglia, neurons, Schwann cells, astrocytes and capillary endothelium. Peripheral nerves also showed extensive lymphohistiocytic infiltration accompanied by axon and myelin sheath degeneration, although it is unclear whether this was a manifestation of the accelerated phase **[7]**.

5. GENETIC ABNORMALITIES

5.1. Gene regulating lysosomal trafficking and study models

The gene responsible for CHS is the lysosome trafficking regulator gene LYST, also known as CHS1 (Chediak-Higashi Syndrome 1) **[23,60]**.

This human gene is located on the long arm of chromosome 1 at position [1q42-43] (**figure 3**) **[15,30]**.

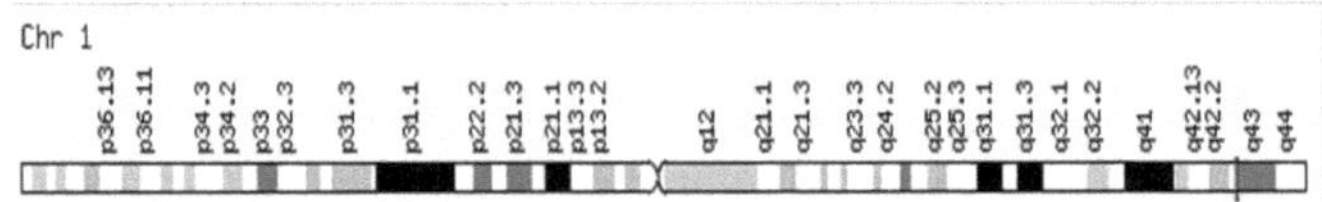

Figure3:Location of the lysosomal traffic regulator gene on chromosome 1 (in red) [61].

It comprises more than 50 exons (**Figure 4**) with an open reading frame of 11,406 bp and codes for a protein of 3,801 amino acids **[42,46]**. Molecular diagnosis is difficult and time-consuming due to the size of the gene **[46]**.

In 1996, the genetic abnormality causing SCH was defined for the first time in rodents and the locus was historically known as beige because of the associated hypopigmentation phenotype. The human homologue of the mouse beige locus then revealed the first mutations causing SCH in humans **[1,41,46]**.

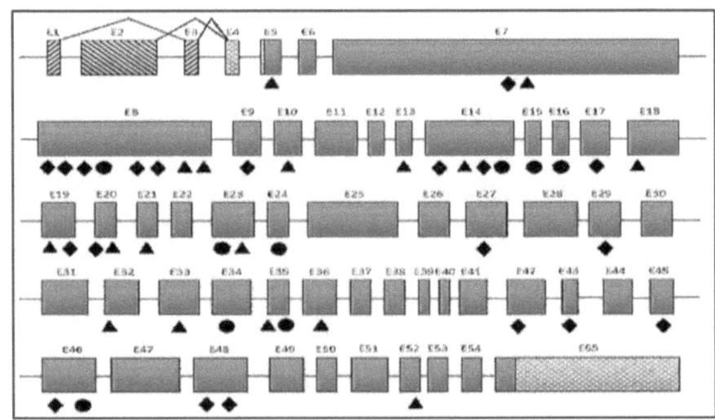

Figure4:Composition of the lysosomal traffic regulator gene [38].

(E:exon)

Similar degrees of identity are observed among the CHS1 genes of humans, rats and cows **[38]**. Genetic linkage studies have shown that LYST is located in a conserved linkage group between human chromosome 1q42- q43 and the Beige region of mouse chromosome 13. The Beige mutant allele was the first mutation in the murine LYST gene to arise spontaneously following insertion of the LINE1 element into an intron of the murine Beige gene producing a premature stop codon. Beige mice on a C57BL/6J background show hypertrophy of lysosomes and lysosome-related organelles, hypopigmentation, and immunodeficiency due to defective cytotoxicity of LTc and NK **[1,23]**.

Other animal species affected by CHS have made it possible to better identify abnormalities in the LYST gene. These species include the cow and the Aleutian mink **[1]**. Feline CHS was observed for the first time in a line of Persian cats and, as in mice, the disease was autosomal recessive and the sentinel presentation was hypopigmentation (**Figure 5**). neutrophil and platelet functions and abnormalities in auditory and ocular pigmentation. Affected cats also have photophobia and pale yellow-green irises, rather than the normal coppery irises of their healthy companions **[60]**.

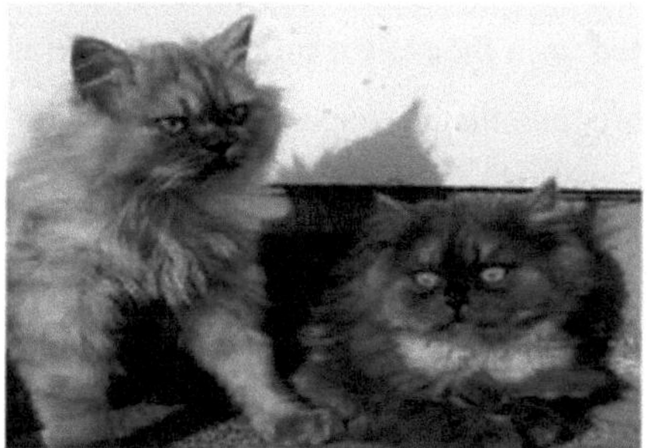

Figure 5: Chediak-Higashiche syndrome in cats aged 5 months[60] The affected cat (left) has a lighter skin tone (hypopigmentation) than its unaffected companion (right).

Although several animal models of CHS have been studied, none has consistently mimicked the human neurological phenotype **[33]**.

5.2. Mutations responsible for disease

Many mutations in the LYST gene have been described in CHS, given its large size. As of 2017, 63 CHS1/LYST mutations have been described, including 31 substitutions (20 nonsense, 11 missense), 19 deletions, nineinsertions and four acceptor splice sites **[6]**.

In 2020, mutations in the LYST gene reached 74. These include missense and nonsense variants, as well as small deletions and insertions in the coding region that have been identified throughout the gene, particularly in the ARM/HEAT, BEACH and WD-40 domains **[15,41,42,62,63]**. Determining the pathogenicity of the new variants poses problems. Bioinformatics prediction tools offer some guidance in determining pathogenicity, but the clinical phenotype is also important in interpreting molecular variations **[1]**.

Most of these mutations are nonsense or null mutations and affect splice sites, leading to the absence of CHS1/LYST protein. These loss-of-function mutations are generally associated with the severe infantile form of CHS, leading to death if left untreated. More attenuated forms described with missense mutations probably encode a partially functional protein **[32,41]**.

In 1996, Nagle et al. identified mutations in three patients. In the first case, a single base deletion at codon 489 caused premature termination at codon 566. The second was a mutation at codon 1103, and the third was a single base duplication at codon 40 **[64]**.

Karim et al. defined two additional frameshift mutations, i.e. a single base insertion at codon 633/634 with a premature stop at codon 638 and a single base deletion at codon 3197 producing a premature stop codon at 3258. They explained that all 3801 amino acids were required for the function of the LYST gene, since the latter mutation resulted in classic severe symptoms of CHS **[65]**.

In 1997, Barbosa et al. identified three additional mutations, namely a single base substitution at nucleotide148 with a premature stop at codon 50, a single base substitution at nucleotide 3085 resulting in termination at codon 1029, and a two-base deletion at nucleotides 3073/3074 with a premature stop codon at 1030 **[66]**.

Consequently, the majority of mutations observed resulted in a reading frame shift with premature termination **[23]**.

In a nationwide survey of 15 CHS patients in Japan, LYST gene analysis was performed in 10 cases. Seven different mutations were detected in seven patients. All of these mutations were frameshift or nonsense mutations, resulting in loss of function of the LYST protein, and the remaining three patients clinically diagnosed with CHS had no mutations in the LYST gene **[28]**.

Karimetal. reported a mutational analysis ofLYST in 21 patients. with CHS. No mutation was found in ten patients, but a heterozygous mutation was found in four patients. It is possible that other responsible genes exist, or that the mutation is located in the introns or in the splicing zones in patients without detected LYST mutations **[67]**.

If no LYST mutation is found, CHS could be caused by dysfunction of genes playing a crucial role in the internalisation of substances and their transport to the perinuclear endocytic recycling compartment **[67]**.

Tables I and II show the LYST variants with the main mutations described in the literature up to the year 2022 for the adult and infantile form, as well as the effect of the anomalies on the LYST protein.

Table I: Regulator gene mutations observed in the adult form of Chediak-Higashi syndrome

Genetic abnormality	Effects on proteinLYST	Reference
c.5784+5G >T	Receptor spliceosome	[68]
c.5996T >A	V1999D	[65]
c.9827_9832del6pb	N3276_T3277del	[58]
c.10127A>G	N3376S	[69]
c.2413delG	E805fsX806	
c.8428G>A	E2810K	[65]
c.4274delT	L1425fsX1426	
c.4361C>A	A1454D	
c.5061T >A	Y1687X	
c.9925G>A	G3309S	[70]
c.1507C>T	R503X	
c.8583G>A	W2861X	[65]
c.148C>T	R50X	[66]
c.3944-3945insC	Q1847fsX1850	[52]
c.575insT	L192FfsX6	[71]
c.575_576insT	L192fsX197	[65]
c.961T >C	C258R	[72]
c.4189T >G	F1397V	[73]
c.4688G>A	R1563H	[65]

c.:codingDNA;del:deletion;ins:insertion;X:codonstop;fsX:frameshift;o:opposite strand; bp: base pair; A: adenine; C: cytosine; G: guanine; T: thymine. Amino acid abbreviations : A: Alanine; R: Arginine; N: Asparagine; D: Aspartate or aspartic acid;C:Cysteine;E:Glutamateorglutamic acid;Q:Glutamine;G:Glycine;L:Leucine;K: Lysine; F: Phenylalanine; S: Serine; T: Threonine; W: Tryptophan; Y: Tyrosine; V: Valine.

Table II: Mutations in the lysosomal traffic regulator gene observed in the infantile form of Chediak-Higashi syndrome

Genetic abnormality	Effect on proteinLYST	Reference
c.1467delG	E489fsX566	[64]
c.1899insA	K633fsX638	[67]
c.9590delA	Y3197fsX3258	
c.3085C>T	Q1029X	[66]
c.2620delT	F874fsX898	[74]
c.10395delA	K3465fsX3467	[65]
c.7060-7066del7pb	L2354fsX2369	[71]
c.7555delT	Y2519fsX2528	[75]
c.9106-9161del56pb	G3036fsX3051	
c.6078C>A	Y2026X	[65]
c.5004delA	G1668fsX1717	[71]
c.5519delC	S1840fsX1842	
c.11102G>T	E3668X	[76]
c.5506C>T	R1836X	[2]
c.7060-1G>A	Acceptor splice	[65]
c.10551_10552del2	Y3517X	
c.2374_2375delGA	D792fsX797	
c.4508C>G	S1483X	
c.2570C>G	S857C	
c.9930delT	F3310fsX3346	
c.1540C>T	R514X	[77]
c.9893delT	F3298fsX3304	
c.3622C>T	Q1208X	[78]
c.10445insCA	V3483fsX3516	[78]
Not specified	R2403X	
c.5317delA	R1773fsX1785	[75]
c.9228ins10bp	K3077fsX3080	
c.118insG	A40fsX63	[79]
c.3073+3074delA	N1025fsX1030	[66]
c.2454delA	K818fsX823	[65]
c.3434-3435insA	H1145fsX1153	
c.4052C>G	S1351X	
c.3944-3945insC	T1315fsX1331	[52]
c.11196-1G>A	Acceptor splice	[65]
c.11362G>A	G3725R	[72]
c.925C>T	R309X	[80]

c.:codingDNA;del:deletion;ins:insertion;X:codonstop;fsX:frameshift;o:opposite strand; bp: base pair; A: adenine; C: cytosine; G: guanine; T: thymine. Amino acid abbreviations : A: Alanine; R: Arginine; N: Asparagine; D: Aspartate or aspartic acid;C:Cysteine;E:Glutamateorglutamic acid;Q:Glutamine;G:Glycine;L:Leucine;K: Lysine; F: Phenylalanine; S: Serine; T: Threonine; W: Tryptophan; Y: Tyrosine; V: Valine.

5.3 Study genetics

Chediak-Higashi syndrome is a rare genetic disorder that is transmitted autosomal recessively. As a result, the parents of sufferers may be heterozygous for the disease (i.e. they carry an abnormal LYST gene). A molecular biology test must be carried out to verify the carrier status of the parents, and siblings of diagnosed cases must be rapidly assessed. This will allow transplantation to take place before complications, particularly the accelerated phase, develop **[11,81]**.
Genetic testing can be performed to assess the status of children if family-specific pathogenic variants are known. In addition, a peripheral blood test may be performed to detect the presence of inclusions in white blood cells **[82]**.
The best time to determine genetic risk and carrier status is before any pregnancy. Preimplantation genetic diagnosis is also an option for those whose LYST pathogenic genes have been identified. DNA banking options should also be offered to sufferers, with extracted DNA, usually from white blood cells, being stored for future use. It is possible that testing and understanding of genes will improve in the future **[82]**.

5.4. Correlation genotype-phenotype

Studies have suggested a correlation between mutation type and clinical phenotype. Patients with mutations resulting in truncated and/or loss-of-function proteins (due to nonsense mutations or frameshifts) are generally symptomatic early in life with highly lethal disease. On the other hand, later and/or milder forms are seen mainly in patients with missense or splice-site mutations **[33,83]**.

However, other studies are to the contrary. Patients with mutations that truncate the protein have shown mild phenotypes, manifesting themselves in adulthood **[12,83]**.
In addition, Kaya et al reported the cases of two siblings who carried identical mutations but had very different clinical severities. This finding suggests that the genotype-phenotype correlation is not always true. Further studies are needed to

better characterise the molecular basis of phenotypic heterogeneity in CHS. It is likely that other factors may act to modulate the phenotype, such as epigenetic markers, other genes involved and different exposure to pathogens **[83]**.

Furthermore, comparison of the cytotoxic function of NKs in CHS patients with mutations found in the ARM/HEAT or BEACH domains of LYST did not reveal any correlation between the degree of NK cytotoxicity and the position of the mutations, but the latter did correlate positively with the size and number of lytic granules in NK cells **[1]**.

Pathogenic variants in the ARM/HEAT domain resulted in a reduced number of lytic granules, but clearly enlarged granules capable of migrating towards the immunological synapse but unable to fuse with the plasma membrane. In contrast, pathogenic variants of the BEACH domain lead to normal or slightly enlarged granules that have altered the polarisation of the immunological synapse. In both cases, exocytosis of lytic granules is impaired, with significantly reduced cytotoxicity **[30]**. We note that the genotype-phenotype correlation within the LYST gene may also play a role in determining certain predilections for specific types of neurological deficiency **[7,59]**.

A genotype-phenotype correlation exists in the two mouse models of CHS. The beige mouse closely reflects the classic form of CHS with dilution of pigments, enlarged granules in several types of cells, including leukocytes, and granulocyte dysfunction, but no neurological manifestations. The second mouse model, LystIng3618/LystIng3618, created by mutagenesis, is homozygous for a missense mutation. This model has a predominant neurological phenotype with blunted pigment dilution, but no immunological defects. It therefore more closely recapitulates the phenotype of the atypical form. Unfortunately, in the case of human CHS, a specific correlation between mutation types and neurological phenotype has not been established **[7,59]**.

6. CLINICAL SIGNS

Characteristic features of CHS include partial oculocutaneous albinism, a tendency to bleed, recurrent infections and neurodegeneration **[1]**.

However, early infections may resolve and not be mentioned by the patient or family members. Bleeding is generally benign and can also be easily overlooked. Finally, albinism is partial and may be very slight or limited to the skin, hair, iris or retina **[83]**.

6.1. Albinism

Broadly speaking, there are three main forms of albinism: oculocutaneous albinism (of which there are seven subtypes), X-linked ocular albinism (AO1) and syndromic albinism (Hermansky-Pudlak syndrome and Chediak-Higashi syndrome). These syndromic forms are accompanied by variable cutaneous and ocular phenotypes and additional symptoms such as haemostasis abnormalities, predisposition to infections and intellectual disability **[55,62,84,85]**.

Partial oculocutaneous albinism is an important feature of CHS, but the degree of pigment dilution varies and may be present normally, partially or absent, and may involve the skin, hair and/or eyes **[15,86]**.

The clinical presentation of CHS is usually a combination of fair skin, silvery hair and variable photosensitivity, in addition to infections **[12]**.

Cutaneous albinism is characterised by hypopigmentation of the skin and dander. Melanocytes are present in the deep layers of the epidermis and hair follicles, but do not produce melanin at all, or only in limited quantities **[84]**.

Hair can be blond, grey or white, and is often distinguished by a silvery or metallic sheen often seen in classic forms of the disease (**Figure 6**) **[6,15]**. Silver and white hair are clinical signs that always require medical examination **[27]**. In addition to the dilution of skin and hair pigments, ocular albinism can be subtle, particularly in people with dark iris pigmentation **[87]**. This ocular albinism is characterised by horizontal or rotational nystagmus, hypopigmentation of the iris with transillumination visible on examination (**Figure 7**), depigmentation of the retina with variable macular transparency, hypoplasia of the fovea and optic nerve, strabismus, variable reduction in visual acuity and photophobia. These defects may be compounded by astigmatism, hyperopia or myopia **[15]**.

Once thought to be an essential criterion for clinical diagnosis, it is now known that some individuals show no signs of oculocutaneous albinism **[1]**.

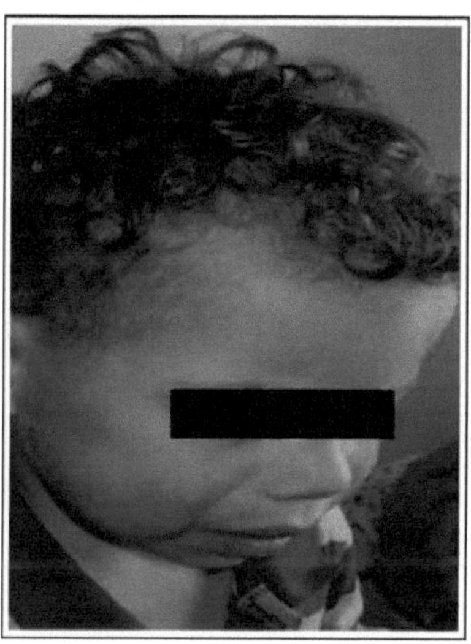

Figure6:Two-year-old child with Chediak-Higashi syndrome showing blond hair and hypopigmentation of the skin [88].

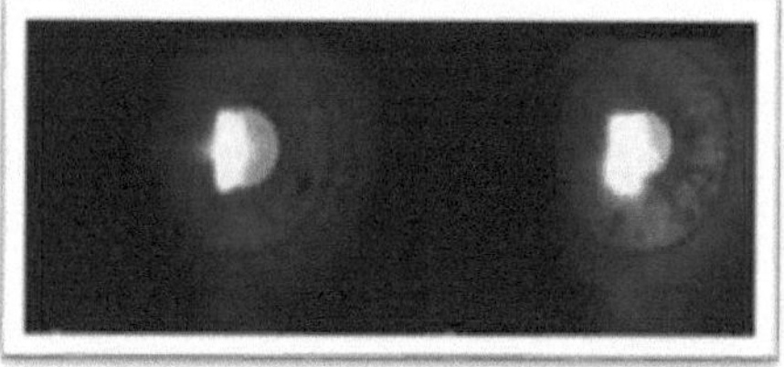

Figure7:Image of a patient with Chediak-Higash syndrome showing transillumination of the iris [1].

6.2. Immunodeficiency and recurrent infections

People with CHS suffer from recurrent and often serious infections, which generally begin in early childhood. Skin infections and upper respiratory tract infections are the most common. They are most often of bacterial and fungal origin. Staphylococcal and streptococcal (pneumococcal and beta-haemolytic) species are the most frequently isolated from these infection sites **[6,54,89]**.

Patients with atypical disease may not show symptoms of unusual or serious infections. Recently, periodontitis has been identified as an important indicator of immune dysfunction in the CHS and may help in making a correct diagnosis. Previous studies have noted that humans and animals (e.g. mink, mice, cattle and cats) with CHS are more likely to develop aggressive periodontitis which does not usually respond to mechanical removal of oral bacterial biofilm and/or antibiotics **[57]**.

The results of one study suggest that patients with classic CHS who have received a graft and patients with atypical CHS are less likely to develop aggressive periodontitis compared with patients with classic CHS who have never received a graft **[57]**.

The presence of recurrent infections in a child with the classic form should arouse suspicion, especially if there is a family history **[25]**.

6.3. Haemorrhagic manifestations

Due to the complexity of platelet dense granule biogenesis, defects in these granules are highly heterogeneous. Isolated forms can be distinguished from syndromic forms. The latter are easier to recognise clinically because of the presence of other signs such as oculocutaneous albinism and immune deficiencies associated with abnormal platelet function **[90,91]**.

Various types of haemorrhage have been described in the CHS, such as epistaxis, bleeding gums and bruising. They are subtle and generally do not require medical intervention **[6,15]**.

However, in the context of trauma or surgery, platelet dysfunction may contribute to prolonged bleeding. Furthermore, in the presence of thrombocytopenia associated with the accelerated phase, the risk of haemorrhage is accentuated **[1,92]**.

6.4.Neurological manifestations

Around 50% of cases develop neurological manifestations **[11]**. They are almost constant in patients who survive long enough **[7,93]**.

Despite progress in improving survival and treating the central features of CHS, neurological deterioration in adult CHS patients has been noted **[94]**.

The central neurological manifestations most commonly encountered during the course of CHS include progressive cognitive decline, intellectual disability, stroke, seizures, coma, parkinsonism and cerebellar ataxia. Peripheral nervous system (PNS) manifestations include peripheral neuropathy, amyotrophy and absence of deep tendon reflexes **[7,15,83]**. In addition, a spastic paraplegia phenotype has rarely been reported in CHS **[95]**. A study of a cohort of patients with classic and atypical CHS showed that in many cases, manifestations of the central nervous system (CNS) appear to precede the clinical signs of peripheral neuropathy. Peripheral neuropathy generally manifests itself in the second or third decade of life **[7]**.

The neurological disease has both developmental and degenerative components. Children may show learning difficulties and behavioural abnormalities in early school age. In late adolescence and early adulthood, patients begin to show progressive degeneration, including absence of deep tendon reflexes, signs of cerebellar dysfunction, peripheral neuropathy, length-dependent neuropathy, diffuse neurogenic abnormalities, weakness, spasticity or Parkinsonian symptoms **[1]**. These changes are due to the long-term progression of the disease despite successful haematopoietic stem cell transplantation **[96]**.

Longitudinal analyses suggest that there is little evidence of cognitive decline in adult CHS patients over several years, but these impairments may be exacerbated in adult patients with a classic form who have already received a transplant. Pediatric patients with CHS who have already received a transplant have had average outcomes, but long-term follow-up analyses are needed to elucidate the trajectory of cognition in this disease **[94]**.

Furthermore, the fact that only adult bone marrow transplant (BMT) recipients developed neuropathy and not BMT children, suggests that the neuropathy is related to a degenerative process and is not related to conditioning regimens with agents given prior to BMT in childhood **[7]**.

Unlike other clinical features, the neurological disease does not allow a distinction to be made between classic and more atypical phenotypes. However, in people with atypical phenotypes, neurological features may dominate the clinical picture, while haematological and immunological features are more subdued **[1].**

Although case reports often include a discussion of impairments in cognition and daily functioning, most do not base these findings on formal neuropsychological tests but rather on academic performance or ability to work. In addition, the relatively small sample sizes in these studies, combined with the lack of longitudinal neuropsychological data, make these studies difficult to generalise **[94]**. Other factors, such as consanguineous parentage and whether or not a patient has received a bone marrow transplant, may be taken into account and may affect cognition which further contributes to the inability to generalise the results of case reports to other patients and also prevents the impact of the disease on cognition from being isolated. It is clear that the cognitive presentation of affected adults is variable, but no study has systematically assessed the neuropsychological phenotype of the disease **[94]**.

Unfortunately, there is no treatment for the neurological component of CHS. One way of discovering potential treatments for the neurodegenerative component of CHS is through mouse genetics. As in humans, mice with mutations in the LYST gene can also develop progressive neurological deficits **[59]**.

6.5. Specific clinical features of the accelerated phase

The accelerated phase, also known as LHH, is the main cause of death in CHS. It occurs in 85% of sufferers and can occur at any age **[1,97-101]**.
Patients with a classic form seem to have a higher risk of developing an accelerated phase, although exceptions have been reported with individuals with atypical forms who accelerate **[33,34,102,103]**.

Although the triggers of this phase remain unclear, infections such as Epstein-Barr virus (EBV) infection and the absence of NK cell function favoured its development **[25]**. The diagnosis of LHH must be based on clinical and biological criteria [1,101]. According to the 2004 guidelines from Henter et al, clinical criteria include fever and splenomegaly (**Figure 8**). In addition, there are other suggestive signs, such as skin rash, jaundice, oedema, pleural or pericardial effusions **[1]**. Stroke-like episodes, cognitive deficits, myositis, ataxia and hypotonia have also been described, almost always during the course of HHH in CHS cases **[83]**.

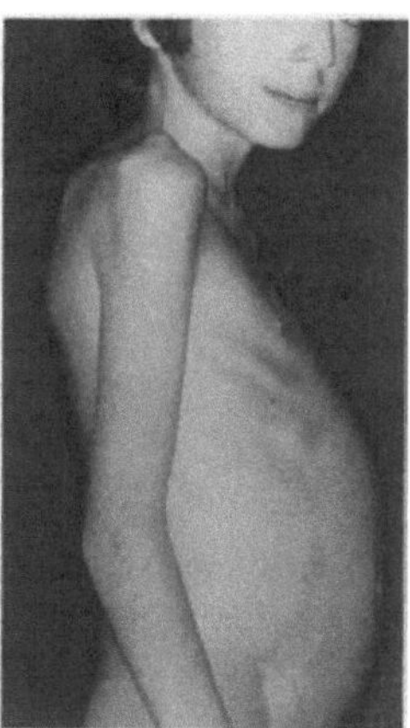

Figure 8: Patient in the accelerated phase of Chediak-Higashi syndrome with marked weight loss and hepatosplenomegaly [104].

7. BIOLOGICAL DIAGNOSIS

Clinical suspicion is confirmed by laboratory evaluation, in particular haematological results **[26]**.

7.1. Haematological diagnosis

7.1.1. Blood count

In CHS, anaemia, thrombocytopenia and/or leukoneutropenia may be present **[1]**. In addition, platelet and leukocyte abnormalities, observed on MGG-stained blood smears or by electron microscopy, can often lead to a diagnosis thanks to the demonstration of specific inclusions (**figures 9, 10 and 11**) probably derived from abnormal fusion between granules **[15,26,40,82,91,102,105]**.

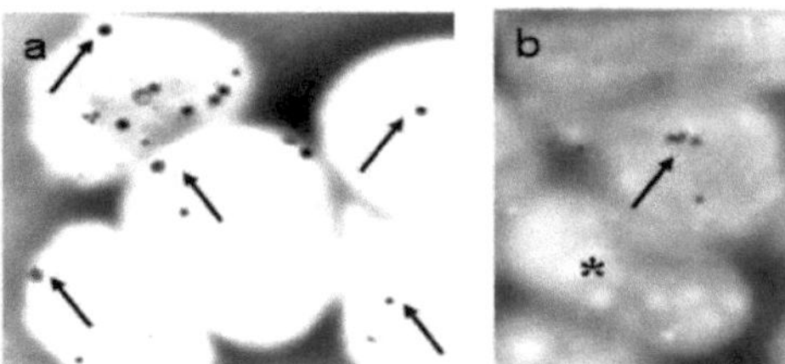

Figure9:Electron microscopy of platelets showing several dense antibodies in control platelets (a), platelets with no dense antibodies and others with a few irregular dense granules in the Chediak-Higashi syndrome patient (b) [30].

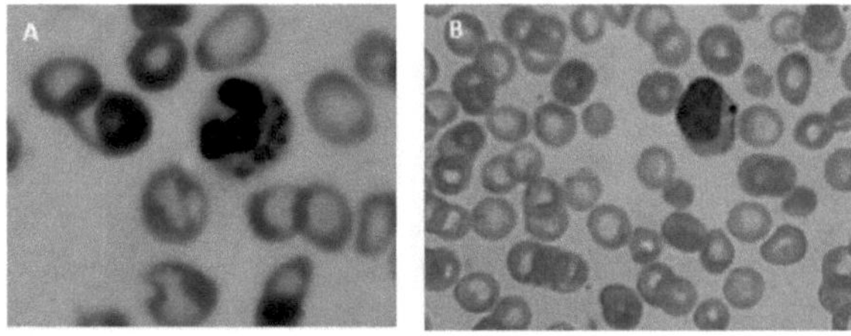

Figure 10 A): Intracytoplasmic inclusions in a neutrophil polynuclear cell in a patient with Chediak-Higashi Syndrome;B):Intracytoplasmic inclusion in a lymphocyte in a patient with Chediak-Higashi Syndrome [59].

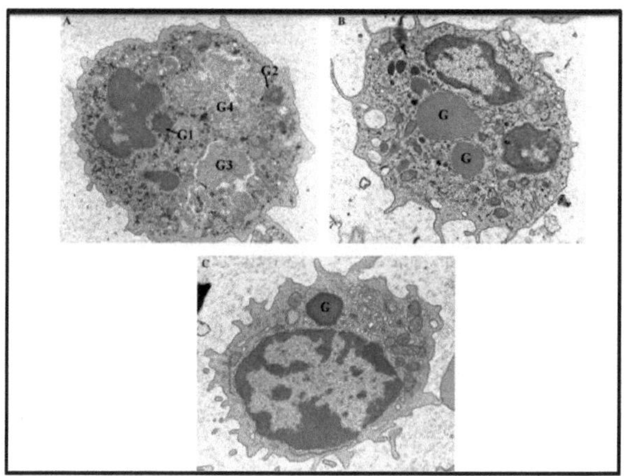

Figure11: Electron micrographs of leukocytes[77].

A) Defined section of a neutrophilic nuclear nucleus (NNN) in a blood sample from a patient with CHS. The cytoplasm is filled with normal-sized organelles, as well as giant lysosomes. Two of the large granules (G1, G2) are intact, another (G3) is beginning to disintegrate, and a fourth (G4) has been transformed into an autophagic vacuole.

B) Thin section of a monocyte from the blood of the same patient. (small granules and two giant granules (G) are present in the cytoplasm.

C) Thin section of a lymphocyte from the blood of the same patient. A giant granule (G) is present in the cytoplasm.

These granules are observed in granulocytes, lymphocytes and rarely in monocytes on smears stained with MGG (May-Grünwald Giemsa), but in certain atypical cases, the presence of these giant granules may be subtle **[7,26,35,58,87,106,107]**. It should also be noted that in acute leukaemias, and rarely in chronic myeloid leukaemias and myelodysplastic syndromes, the presence of giant cytoplasmic inclusions has been observed in myeloblasts or other myeloid precursors, resembling those observed in CHS, hence the name: pseudo-Chediak-Higashi granules **[10,25,108-111]**.

7.1.2. Myelogram

It is characterised by the presence of abnormal cytoplasmic inclusions in lymphocytes, polymorphonuclear cells and bone marrow precursors **(Figure 12)** **[26]**. Ultra-structural studies show that granules contain giant lysosomes and fibrillar structures in myeloid cells **[96]**.

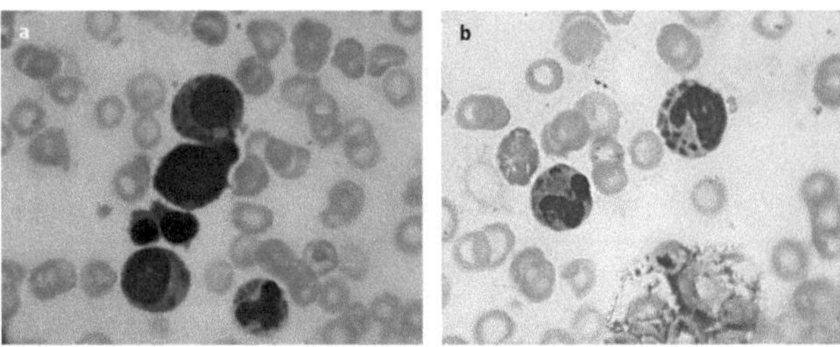

Figure12:Abnormal intracytoplasmic inclusions in granular precursors and neutrophils characteristic of Chediak-Higashi syndrome in a May-Grünwald Giemsa stained bone marrow smear from a nine month old patient [112].

The myelogram should also be examined for the presence of haemophagocytosis characteristic of the transition to the accelerated phase **[1]**.

7.2. Anatomopathological examination

Microscopic examination reveals cytoplasmic inclusions in fibroblasts, neurons, astrocytes, choroid plexus epithelium, Schwann cells and blood vessel endothelial cells, as well as degenerative changes in axons and myelin sheaths. Degenerative changes in axons and myelin sheaths have also been noted **[96,105]**.CHS mouse models show neuronal accumulation of giant lysosomes and intra-cytoplasmic inclusions in Purkinje cells of the cerebellum and motor cortex **[96]**.

Microscopic examination of the hair may also reveal agglomerated melanin granules, larger than those seen in normal hair (**Figure 13**) **[96,113]**. However, examination of the skin can be a useful complementary study in cases where the distribution of pigments in the hair shaft does not support the diagnosis **[87]**. Indeed, it shows giant melanosomes in keratinocytes and melanocytes, which can be used as a laboratory tool for differential diagnosis with other disorders of partial albinism **[96]**. It would be interesting to carry out this test in patients with fair skin and blond hair **[87,114]**.

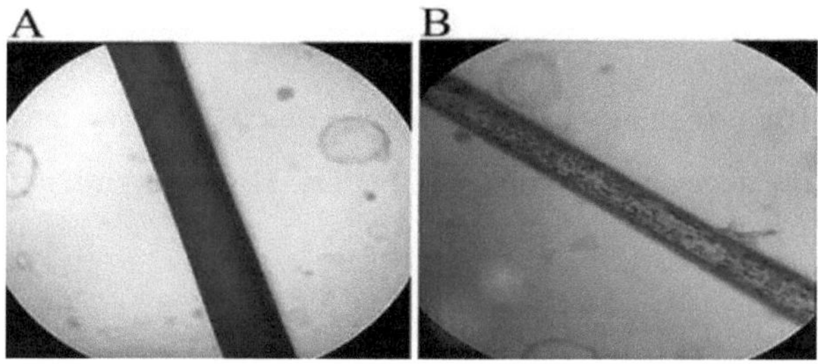

Figure13:Microscopicaspectofhair:Abnormal;B:inChediak-Higashi syndrome [6].

7.3. Prenatal diagnosis

As the disease is autosomal recessive, it is recommended that the patient's parents be screened by examining the blood smears and bone marrow smears. Prenatal diagnosis is possible by studying lysosomes in amniotic fluid cells and leukocytes in foetal blood **[11]**.

7.4. Biological diagnosis of the accelerated phase This phase is due to the appropriate stimulation of macrophages in the bone marrow and lymphoid organs, leading to phagocytosis of blood cells (**Figure 14**) and the production of a large number of pro-inflammatory cytokines **[15,34,98,115-117]**.

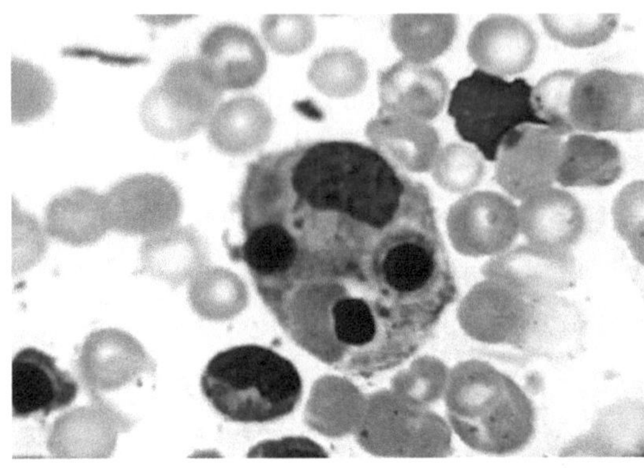

Figure 14: Hemophagocytic hemophagocytic cell on bone marrow smear during the accelerated phase of Chediak-Higashi syndrome [112].

According to the 2004 guidelines from Henter et al, the biological signs of LHH include cytopenias affecting two or three cell lineages (haemoglobin < 90g/L; platelets < 100G/L; neutrophils < 1G/L), hypertri- glyceridaemia > 3 mmol/L and/or hypofibrinogenemia <1.5g/L, haemophagocytosis, low NK cell activity, hyperferritinaemia>500g/L, and elevated levels of soluble interleukin-2 receptor (sCD25>2400U/mL) **[1]**.

Hypoproteinemia, hyponatremia, elevated transaminases and lactate dehydrogenase may be present. Diffuse lymphohistiocytic infiltration is also seen in the liver, spleen, bone marrow, lymph nodes and central nervous system **[1]**. Immunoglobulin and complement levels are usually normal **[96]**.

8. NEUROIMAGING

Neurological signs may be the reason why these patients seek medical attention **[83]**. Brain imaging is not initially revealing, but over time cerebellar and/or cerebral atrophy may develop **[1]**.

These signs are mainly associated with involvement of the posterior fossae. Neuroimaging shows septomeningeal and perivascular cellular infiltration with scattered microscopic granulomas and microglial nodules in the brainstem, cerebellum, spinal cord and peripheral nerves **[96]**.

Interestingly, on MRI (Magnetic Resonance Imaging), the posterior fossa shows structural variability with an acute tentorium, supporting the theory that the development of the posterior fossa is affected (**Figure 15**) **[1]**.

Only a small number of neuroimaging studies of Chédiak-Higashi syndrome have been documented, and the brain MRI features reported are few, inconsistent and extremely variable. One case reported during the accelerated phase of the disease showed supra- and infratentorial lesions with significant involvement of the brainstem and cerebellum **[96]**.

Herman and Lee described supratentorial neoplasm-like contrast-enhancing masses predominantly in the left frontal white matter with mass effect in a 4-year-old boy who had presented with right-sided weakness, lethargy and fever for several weeks during the accelerated phase of the disease. An increase in T2 signal intensity without contrast enhancement was demonstrated in the periventricular and corona radiata regions in a 10-year-old girl 4 months after the onset of acute weakness in the lower extremities with subsequent progression to the trunk and upper limbs. Cerebellar atrophy was reported in a 20-year-old woman several months after the onset of tremors of the upper limbs, tongue and mandible. Neuro Similar images have been reported in patients with familial haemophagocytic lymphohistiocytosis. The observations are non-specific **[96]**.

According to Rego et al, three main patterns of parenchymal involvement can be identified: diffuse, focal and mixed diffuse/focal. Cerebral atrophy at the time of diagnosis was a common finding **[96]**.

In patients with CHS, the central and peripheral systems may show varying degrees of infiltration by lymphocytes and histiocytes: cellular infiltration may be found in the leptomeninges, choroid plexuses, intraprenchymal blood vessels, particularly venules, and in cranial and spinal nerve roots. Less commonly, focal aggregates of histiocytes and lymphocytes may give rise to scattered microscopic granulomas or microglial nodules **[96]**.

Neuroimaging plays a vital role in assessing CNS changes in AP, particularly in atypical forms where characteristic signs such as fever and hepatosplenomegaly may be absent. As reactivation during treatment is frequent, neuroimaging is essential for follow-up **[96]**.

In a patient from northern Finland whose diagnosis of CHS was confirmed at the age of 2, allogeneic OMT was performed shortly after diagnosis. At the age of 30, MRI showed global cerebral and cerebellar atrophy, as well as a decrease in the volume of the posterior corpus callosum. The lateral ventricles were also dilated, with no evidence of hydrocephalus. No abnormalities were evident in the spinal cord (**Figure 16) [93]**.

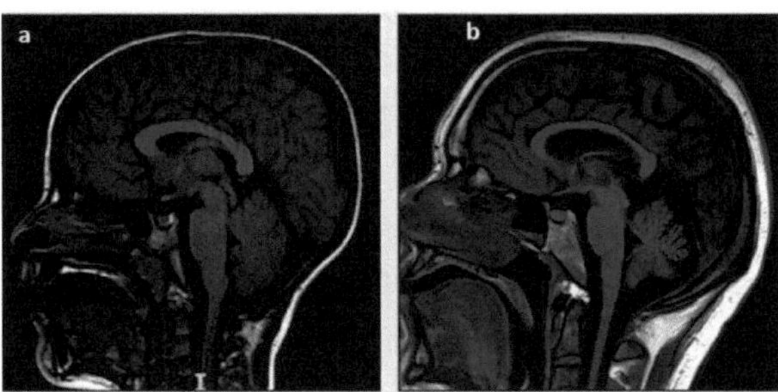

Figure 15: Magnetic resonance imaging showing posterior fossa atrophy in a child (a) and cerebellar and cerebral atrophy in an adult (b) [1].

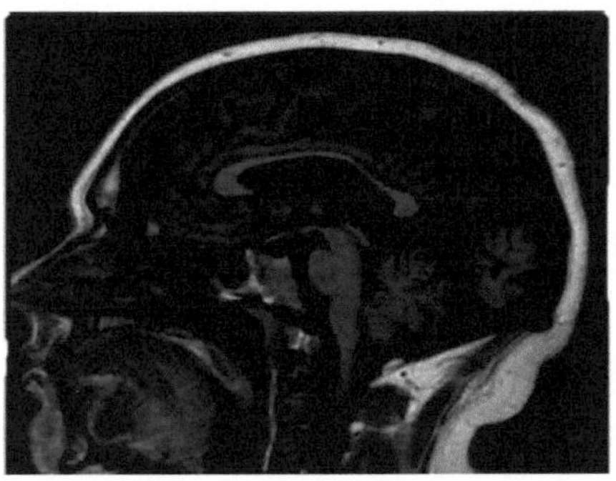

Figure 16: Magnetic resonance imaging showing global cerebral and cerebellar atrophy, and a decrease in the volume of the posterior corpus callosum [93].

9. DIFFERENTIAL DIAGNOSIS

Like CHS, other genetic diseases are associated with oculocutaneous albinism. However, the large patho- gnomonic inclusions of Chediak-Higashi disease are absent. In addition, the diagnosis must combine all the clinical, biological, histological and genetic components **[40,42]**.

Differential diagnoses include Griscelli syndrome (GS) and Elejalde syndrome, which are characterised by silvery hair, pigment abnormalities and central nervous system dysfunction.Hair microscopy can aid diagnosis: in CHS, it shows evenly distributed aggregates of melanin of regular diameter, whereas in Griscelli syndrome, the melanin granules are large and mainly found in the medullary area **[25]**. The distribution of pigment in the skin of patients with CHS and GS correlates with that observed in the hair. Therefore, skin biopsy can be a useful complementary study in cases where hair shaft pigmentation has not been observed **[87]**.

On the other hand, only CHS and Griscelli syndrome type 2 (GS2) have been reported to cause HHL. A key finding in differentiating these two entities is the absence of giant cytoplasmic granules in G2S. Neurological manifestations were thought to be uncommon in G2S, but are in fact reported in 67% of patients. Seizures and cranial nerve palsies are the most common abnormalities **[83]**.

Elejalde's syndrome has normal immunological function and capillary microscopy reveals small and large, irregularly distributed aggregates of melanin **[6]**. Hermansky-Pudlak syndrome (HPS) should also be considered in the differential diagnosis, as it is associated with oculocutaneous albinism, platelet storage pool deficiency and, in some subtypes, immunodeficiency **[6]**.

The differentiation factor is that SG and SHP do not have abnormal granules in neutrophils **[1]**.

Cross syndrome is also characterised by hypopigmentation, CNS involvement such as developmental delay and ocular anomalies. Endosomal adaptor p14 deficiency syndrome includes short stature, partial albinism, congenital neutropenia and lymphoid deficiency.neutrophils have azurophilic granules and abnormal microbicidal functions ofphagosomes.this contrasts with t h e giant inclusions seen in CHS neutrophils **[1,15]**.

Familial haemophagocytic lymphohistiocytosis (FHHL) is an autosomal recessive disorder caused by mutation of one of five genes [FHL1-FHL5] corresponding to the five subtypes of the disease. Symptoms include prolonged fever, hepatosplenomegaly and neurological abnormalities. The disease manifests itself in the first few months or in utero. Symptoms may also appear later in childhood or in adulthood **[1,15]**.

10. THERAPEUTIC MANAGEMENT

The management of CHS can be classified as follows: symptomatic management of complications associated with the disease (cutaneous, infectious, haemorrhagic, neurological, etc.), treatment of the accelerated phase or LHH and haematopoietic stem cell transplantation (HSCT). HSCT has been recognised as the most effective treatment for the haematological and immune deficiencies caused by CHS, but it cannot improve neurological dysfunction. Rapid diagnosis of CHS facilitates early therapeutic intervention before the development of LHH, thus preventing permanent damage caused by lymphocytic infiltration of vital organs **[7]**.

10.1. Symptomatic treatment

To manage signs of oculocutaneous albinism, sunglasses should be worn to protect sensitive eyes from UV rays and refractive error correction can be performed to improve visual acuity. In addition, people should apply sunscreen to prevent skin cancer and sun damage. The degree of protection depends on the severity of the hypopigmentation **[15]**.

To manage infectious complications, the patient must be protected as far as possible from exposure to infectious agents, and appropriate vaccinations must be administered. In the case of bacterial infections, the rapid and intensive use of antibiotics is essential. However, the use of generalised antibiotic prophylaxis before dental or invasive procedures is controversial, but should be considered in people with compromised immune systems and neutropenia **[15]**.

Other modes of treatment have been proposed, including the administration of vitamin C during the stable phase to normalise the bactericidal activity of neutrophils and high-dose methylprednisolone, with or without splenectomy **[118,119]**. Oral infections may present an increased risk of systemic infection in immunocompromised patients, hence the importance of regular dental care to control or prevent infections **[120]**.With regard to the management of bleeding complications, a platelet transfusion may be necessary in the event of serious trauma or major haemorrhage. Before any invasive procedure, desmopressin should be administered intravenously for 30 minutes to help control bleeding. Non-steroidal anti-inflammatory drugs should also be avoided as they can exacerbate bleeding tendencies **[15]**. Currently, there is no effective targeted therapy to alleviate the permanent damage to the nervous system in CHS. With the exception of one case report in which prednisolone was used to treat peripheral neuropathy. Comprehensive rehabilitation and orthoses can provide substantial benefit for people with significant peripheral nervous system involvement and there is a symptomatic response to L- Dopa for patients with parkinsonism **[7]**. As symptoms are progressive in nature, rehabilitation should be started for elderly patients as early as possible in the course of the disease **[15]**. Overall, PNS manifestations are less debilitating than CNS manifestations but may provide a practical method of monitoring future treatments **[7]**. While the majority of early-onset survivors require special support for learning and education, the special education plan must be based on a detailed neuropsychological and neuropsychiatric examination. Learning disabilities in these children may be linked to visual impairments which are rare in the general population and require specific rehabilitation strategies. In addition, (neuro)psychiatric problems are not necessarily present **[93]**.

10.2. Haematopoietic stem cell allograft

Genetic testing is necessary for diagnosis and for allogeneic haematopoietic stem cell transplantation (HSCT), which is the only curative treatment for CHS **[1,6,121,122]**.

In patients with the classic form of CHS, this treatment corrects the immune and haematological defects linked to lysosomal transport, can prevent LHH or the 'accelerated phase' and allows survival into adulthood by considerably reducing the infectious complications of the disease. It should be performed as soon as the diagnosis is established, before the development of the accelerated phase, but the ideal time is not known, given the heterogeneity of the expression of the disease. If signs of accelerated phase are evident, haemophagocytosis should be brought into remission before transplantation **[1,7,12,15]**.

In an Eapen report, nine CHS patients receiving allogeneic HSCT died early, six of whom had persistent disease and received PA transplantation **[89]**. Successful transplantation has been shown to be more common in people whose donors were compatible with the HLA system **[7]**. However, the alternative of transplantation from a non-compatible donor can be proposed as a valid option in the absence of a compatible donor in the family **[93,123-125]**.

HSCT has increased the overall 5-year survival rate to over 50%. However, it does not appear to prevent the neurodegenerative process associated with this disease. Indeed, like patients with the atypical form, patients with the classic form of CHS who have received HSCT later develop similar neurological complications in the PNS and CNS **[7]**.

Tardieu reported three patients who survived for 20 years after haematopoietic stem cell transplantation. These cases had progressively severe central nervous system symptoms including balance abnormalities, tremor, intellectual deficit, dementia, peripheral neuropathy and cerebellar atrophy **[6,104]**. Data have also been published in India by Uppuluri et al. in 2017 on children undergoing haplo-identical HSCT with post-transplant cyclophosphamide with survival in 6 of 8 children in their cohort. However, active infections at the time of transplantation are associated with poorer survival and an increased risk of mortality **[126]**.

Umbilical cord blood (UCB) has become an important alternative source of haematopoietic stem cells for patients with haematological diseases. Five-year survival was higher in children receiving HLA-matched SCO transplants (60%), and 5-year survival after transplants of SCO mismatched for one or two antigens was similar to that of bone marrow transplants **[89]**. In recent years, the absence or decrease in the intensity of CD107a protein measured on the surface of cells by flow cytometry has shown high sensitivity and specificity for the diagnosis of primary granule exocytosis disorder, which has been verified in CHS patients with a lack of LTc cytotoxicity. These patients are an indication for early TCSH because of the high risk of developing LHH. Further research should confirm these results, and propose approaches to significantly improve the effect of treatment **[6]**.

10.3. Specific treatment of the accelerated phase

Management of the accelerated phase is the same as for primary forms of LHH and allows remission to be established until definitive treatment can be obtained with HSCT **[1,124,127-129]**.

The first prospective international treatment protocol for LHH was introduced in 1994, followed by the 2004 LHH treatment protocol, which recommends eight weeks' induction therapy with corticosteroids, etoposide (VP16) and cyclosporine A **[6]**.

Intrathecal therapy with methotrexate and prednisone is limited to patients with signs of disease progression in the nervous system. after two weeks of systemic treatment, or in patients with worsening or non-improving cerebrospinal fluid pleocytosis **[6]**.

Around 75% of individuals achieve remission after eight weeks. Relapses are not uncommon, and response to treatment declines over time **[15]**.

In recent decades, a growing understanding of the underlying biological mechanisms of LHH has led to standardised treatment and management protocols, resulting in improved survival **[25,130]**.

A case study of a nine-month-old patient diagnosed with CHS in the accelerated phase presented with a rapid progression of LHH symptoms. He was treated with high dose dexamethasone and etoposide. Cyclosporine A was administered two weeks later due to poor compliance. His temperature fell within 72 hours and normalised within seven days. All blood tests returned to normal about 3-4 weeks later **[6]**. Etoposide (VP16) is a cytotoxic agent that acts on both the mitotic spindle and topoisomerases II. Although non-specific, it has a particular tropism for the monocyte-macrophage lineage. Its efficacy in HHH has long been reported, and validated by several protocols. Its superiority to other immunomodulatory treatments (polyvalent immunoglobulins, cyclosporine) has been demonstrated at least in EBV-induced HCL **[131,132]**. Furthermore, in this study, early administration of VP16 influenced long-term survival (90% vs 56% for delayed administration). Etoposide is therefore the reference treatment for HCL in combination with corticosteroids **[131,132]**. A meta-analysis carried out in China showed that of 29 patients with CHS and LHH, 9 received chemotherapy with a 100% improvement rate; however, of the 20 other patients who received only standard antibiotic treatment, 11 died **[133]**. The age of onset of the disease, the course, and the presence of LHH are critical factors in determining whether chemotherapy should be performed **[6]**.

In certain specific cases, other treatments may be discussed [133]. Polyvalent immunoglobulins have shown some efficacy in HCL secondary to viral infections. However, they are only fully effective in episodes without signs of severity. Specific inhibition of T lymphocyte activation and proliferation by cyclosporine means that treatment of immune deficiency with HSCT can be deferred without prolonged exposure to leukaemogenic products. In the case of persistent bone marrow failure, Kaito et al. have proposed a combination of anti-lymphocyte serum and cyclosporine A **[131]**.

To improve survival, studies have focused on the use of new therapies to reduce inflammation in HCL. Among the agents being tested is ruxolitinib, a potent inhibitor of the Janus Kinase (JAK) pathway and the Signal Transducer and Activation of Transcription (STAT) pathway, which functions downstream of many LHH-associated cytokines **[134,135]**.

Another study suggests that nivolumab achieves durable control of LHH associated with EBV infection with tolerable toxicity **[136]**.

In refractory or persistent cases of LHH, salvage treatments are used such as antithymocyte immunoglobulins, alemtuzumab as well as other biological agents including rituximab (particularly effective in EBV infections), daclizumab, infliximab, tocilizumab, TNF alpha inhibitors, JAK inhibitors, IVIg, and the anti-gamma interferon antibody: Emapalumab **[137-141]**.

10.4. Gene therapy

The large size of the LYST coding sequence (around 11 kb) represents a major technical obstacle to the development of a gene therapy application for CHS. Even with the recombinant vector of the adeno-associated virus (AAV), which has recently become an attractive approach for many genes, the insert size limit of 5 kb poses a challenge. In addition, the development of a unified approach, given the distribution of pathogenic mutations along the entire length of the coding region **[1]**.

11. PROGNOSIS AND SURVIVAL

CHS is potentially fatal, but HSCT can improve the prognosis. This highlights the need for early identification of affected children **[25,116,142]**. Up to 90% of affected individuals die at a young age from recurrent infections or LHH unless bone marrow transplantation is performed **[15,32]**.

Because it is very difficult to treat, LHH is the most serious complication of SCH. It is associated with a poor prognosis and is the most frequent cause of mortality **[143]**. Without bone marrow transplantation, less than 10% of patients with CHS survive beyond childhood. These patients, whose diagnosis has been confirmed by molecular genotyping, have attenuated clinical features of the disease and can survive into adulthood without haematopoietic cell transplantation and without signs of LHH **[94]**.

A retrospective review of 35 cases of HSCT in patients with CHS reported an overall 5-year survival of 62% **[6]**. Analysis of patients who underwent the HLH-94 protocol indicated that the prognosis without treatment was poor, with a median survival of 1-2 months **[6,25]**.

Bone marrow transplantation is the only curative treatment, if carried out at an early stage. However, there is a risk of several complications, including serious infections and thrombotic microangiopathy, as well as graft-versus-host disease. The bone marrow transplant patient is susceptible to bacterial and fungal infections in the first month after transplantation, due to leukopenia and mucosal damage. The patient continues to have reduced immunity for at least two years and may develop pneumonia, meningitis, cytomegalovirus or herpes zoster infection. The decision as to whether a bone marrow transplant is warranted before the onset of the accelerated phase is therefore incredibly complicated **[115,143]**.

CONCLUSION

CHS (Chediak-Higashi syndrome) is a rare disease characterised by oculocutaneous albinism, mild haemorrhagic diathesis, recurrent infections and neurological dysfunction. The diagnosis is often made by microscopic observation of giant pathognomonic inclusions in leukocytes. Patients with the classic form of the disease are very likely to develop potentially fatal haemophagocytic lymphohistiocytosis (HHL) at an early age, associated with lymphoproliferative infiltration of the reticuloendothelial system and bone marrow.However, those with the atypical form survive into adulthood, mainly developing neurological symptoms. CHS is caused by mutations in the lysosomal trafficking regulator (LYST) gene, which disrupt the formation, transport and fusion of intracellular vesicles. This may explain the characteristics of giant granules in various cell types, including melanocytes and myeloid cells, which are the main diagnostic feature of CHS. To date, 74 pathogenic mutations of LYST in the CHS have been recorded. Bone marrow transplantation is the only curative treatment if carried out at an early stage. Peripheral blood and bone marrow examinations are therefore very important for diagnosis and appropriate management. As CHS is a monogenic disease, it is a good candidate for studies using induced pluripotent stem cells (iPSCs) to better understand the cellular and molecular mechanisms of the disease. In addition, the creation of a drug discovery platform based on iPSCs will make it possible to find better high-throughput treatment options.

REFERENCES

1. Sharma P, Nicoli ER, Serra-Vinardell J, Morimoto M, Toro C, Malicdan MC, et al. Chediak-Higashi syndrome: A review of the past, present, and future. Drug Discov Today Dis Models. 2020;31:31-6.

2. Kalra S, Khera S, Sharma A, Daryani H, Singh V. Chediak Higashi syndromewithacutekidneyinjury:Answers.PediatrNephrol.2022Jan 18.doi:10.1007/s00467-021-05414-z.Onlineaheadofprint.

3. Huang S, Sun HQ, Li HX, Wang LJ. Chediak Higashi syndrome with cytotoxic T-cell lymphoma: a case report. Zhonghua Xue Ye Xue Za Zhi. 2020;41:1051.

4. Meng J, Wang H, Qian X, Miao H, Zhu X, Yu Y, et al. Identification of a novel CHS1/LYST variant in a Chinese pedigree affected with Chediak- Higashi syndrome. ZhonghuaYi XueYi Chuan Xue Za Zhi. 2020;37:441-4.

5. Feizi M, Rajavi Z, Khorshidifar M, Torkian P, Rahimi F. Acute transient sixth nerve palsy in chediak-higashi syndrome. J Pediatr Ophthalmol Strabismus. 2018;55:e22-5.

6. Wu XL, Zhao XQ, Zhang BX, Xuan F, Guo HM, Ma FT. A novel frameshift mutation of Chediak-Higashi syndrome and treatment in the accelerated phase. Braz J Med Biol Res. 2017;50:e5727.

7. Lehky TJ, Groden C, Lear B, Toro C, Introne WJ. Peripheral nervous system manifestations of Chediak-Higashi disease: PNS Manifestations of CHD. Muscle Nerve. 2017;55:359-65.

8. Mozafari R, Rajabnia M, Naleini SN. Chediak-Higashi Syndrome. Arch Iran Med. 2019;22:673-4.

9. Singh A, Jindal AK, Indla R, Sharma P, Varma N, Rawat A. Importance of morphology in the era of molecular biology: lesson learnt from a case of Chediak-Higashi Syndrome. Indian J Hematol Blood Transfus. 2021;37:517-9.

10. YinJ,ZhuS,LuoY,LinZ,ChenY. AcutemyeloidleukaemiawithAuer rods within pseudo-Chédiak-Higashi granules. Br J Haematol. 2020;188:9.

11. Jaiswal P, Yadav YK, Bhasker N, Kushwaha R. Accelerated phase of Chediak-Higashi syndrome at initial presentation: a case report of an uncommon occurrence in a rare disorder. J Clin Diagn Res. 2015;9:ED13- 4.

12. Gomaa NS, Lee JY, El Sharkawy A, El Chazli YF, Hassab HM, Doghaim NN, et al. Genetic analysis in Egyptian patients with Chediak-Higashi syndrome reveals new LYST mutations. Clin Exp Dermatol. 2019;44:814-7.

13. JanniniP,PintolimaFX,HubnerfrancaH,TrictaDF,TannosD. About 3 cases of leukocyte anomaly identical to that described by B'eguez-C'esar, Steinbrinck, Chediak, Higashi and Sato. Sangre (Barc). 1963;13:138-59.

14. Bharti S, Bhatia P, Bansal D, Varma N. The accelerated phase of chediak-higashi syndrome: the importance of hematological evaluation. Turk J Hematol. 2013;30:85-7.

15. AjitkumarA,YarrarapuSN,RamphulK. ChediakHigashiSyndrome. TreasureIsland,FL:StatPearlsPublishing;2021.

16. Chediak MM. New leukocyte anomaly of constitutional and familial character. Rev Hematol. 1952;7:362-7.

17. HigashiO. Congenitalgigantismof peroxidasegranules;the first case ever reported of qualitative abnormity of peroxidase. Tohoku J Exp Med. 1954;59:315-32.

18. Sato A. Chediak and Higashi's disease: probable identity of a new leukocytal anomaly (Chediak) and congenital gigantism of peroxidase granules (Higashi). Tohoku J Exp Med. 1955;61:201-10.

19. Page AR, Berendes H, Warner J, Good RA. The Chediak-Higashi syndrome. Blood. 1962;20:330-43.

20. Kritzler RA, Terner JY, Lindenbaum J, Magidson J, Williams R, Presig R, et al. Chediak-Higashi syndrome. cytologic and serum lipid observations in a case and family. Am J Med. 1964;36:583-94.

21. Lutzner MA, Lowrie CT, Jordan HW. Giant granules in leukocytes of the beige mouse. J Hered. 1967;58:299-300.

22. Oliver C, Essner E. Distribution of anomalous lysosomes in the beige mouse: a homologue of Chediak-Higashi syndrome. J Histochem Cytochem. 1973;21:218-28.

23. Introne W, Boissy RE, Gahl WA. Clinical, molecular, and cell biological aspectssofChediak-Higashisyndrome.MolGenetMetab.1999;68:283-303.

24. Griscelli C, Virelizier JL. Bone marrow transplantation in a patient with Chédiak-Higashi Syndrome. Birth Defects Orig Artic Ser. 1983;19:333-4.

25. CarneiroIM,RodriguesA,PinhoL,de JesusNunes-SantosC, deBarros Dorna M, Moschione Castro AP,and al. Chediak-Higashi syndrome:Lessonsfromle-centrecaseseries.AllergolImmunopathol (Madr). 2019;47:598-603.

26. Lozano ML, Rivera J, Sánchez-Guiu I, Vicente V. Towards the targeted management of Chediak-Higashi syndrome. Orphanet J Rare Dis. 2014;9:132.

27. Gironi LC, Zottarelli F, Savoldi G, Notarangelo LD, Basso ME, Ferrero I, et al. Congenital hypopigmentary disorders with multiorgan impairment: a case report and an overview on gray hair syndromes. Medicina. 2019;55:78.

28. Nagai K, Ochi F, Terui K, Maeda M, Ohga S, Kanegane H, et al. Clinical characteristics and outcomes of Chediak-Higashi syndrome: A nationwide survey of Japan: Chediak-Higashi Syndrome in Japan. Pediatr Blood Cancer. 2013;60:1582-6.

29. Yamada T, Chen-Yoshikawa TF, Oh S, Ito-Taniguchi R, Gochi F, Sato M, et al. Living-donor lung transplantation after bone marrow transplantation for Chediak-Higashi Syndrome. Ann Thorac Surg. 2017;103:e281-3.

30. Toro C, Nicoli ER, Malicdan MC, Adams DR, Introne WJ. Chediak-Higashi Syndrome. In: Adam MP, Ardinger HH, Pagon RA, Wallace SE, Bean LJ, Gripp KW, et al, eds. GeneReviews® . Seattle, WA: University of Washington; 2022.

31. National Organization for Rare Disorders. Chediak Higashi Syndrome. [Online]. 2018 [Accessed 05/01/2022], Available from URL: https://rarediseases.org/rare-diseases/chediak-higashi-syndrome/

32. deAlmeida HL, Kiszewski AE, Vicentini Xavier T, Pirolli F, Antônio Suita de Castro LA. Ultrastructural aspects of hairs of Chediak-Higashi syndrome. J Eur Acad Dermatol Venereol. 2018;32:e227-9.

33. Serra-Vinardell J, Sandler MB, Pak E, Zheng W, Dutra A, Introne W, et al. Generation and characterization of four Chediak-Higashi Syndrome (CHS) induced pluripotent stem cell (iPSC) lines. Stem Cell Res. 2020;47:101883.

34. Cetinkaya PG, Cagdas D, Gumruk F, Tezcan I. Hemophagocytic lymphohistiocytosis in patients with primary immunodeficiency. J Pediatr Hematol Oncol. 2020;42:e434-9.

35. Yarnell DS, Roney JC, Teixeira C, Freitas MI, Cipriano A, Leuschner P, et al. Diagnosis of Chediak Higashi disease in a 67‐year old woman. Am J Med Genet. 2020;182:3007-13.

36. Delevoye C, Marks MS, Raposo G. Lysosome-related organelles as functional adaptations of the endolysosomal system. Curr Opin Cell Biol. 2019;59:147-58.

37. Lattao R, Rangone H, Llamazares S, Glover DM. Mauve/LYST limits fusion of lysosome-related organelles and promotes centrosomal recruitment of microtubule nucleating proteins. Dev Cell. 2021;56:1000- 13.

38. XuX,ShenW. Chediak-HigashiSyndrome. [Online].2019 [Accessed

05/01/2022], available à the URL:
http://atlasgeneticsoncology.org/Kprones/ChediakHigashiID10128.html

39. Steffens A, Jakoby M, Hülskamp M. Physical, functional and genetic interactions between the BEACH domain protein SPIRRIG and LIP5 and SKD1 and its role in endosomal trafficking to the vacuole in arabidopsis. Front Plant Sci. 2017;8:1969.

40. Zamani R, Shahkarami S, Rezaei N. Primary immunodeficiency associated with hypopigmentation: A differential diagnosis approach. Allergol Immunopathol (Madr). 2021;49:178-90.

41. Boluda-Navarro M, Ibáñez M, Liquori A, Franco-Jarava C, Martínez-Gallo M, Rodríguez-Vega H, et al. Case Report: partial uniparental disomy unmasks a novel recessive mutation in the LYST gene in a patient with a severe phenotype of Chédiak-Higashi Syndrome. Front Immunol. 2021;12:625591.

42. Song Y, Dong Z, Luo S, Yang J, Lu Y, Gao B, et al. Identification of a compound heterozygote in LYST gene: a case report on Chediak-Higashi syndrome. BMC Med Genet. 2020;21:4.

43. Introne W, Boissy RE, Gahl WA. Clinical, Molecular, and CellBiological Aspects of Chediak-Higashi Syndrome. Mol Genet Metab. 1999;68:283- 303.

44. Zbinden JC, Mirhaidari GJM, Blum KM, Musgrave AJ, Reinhardt JW, Breuer CK, etal. Thelysosomal trafficking regulator isnecessaryfor normal wound healing. Wound Repair Regen. 2022;30:82-99.

45. Parenti G, Medina DL, Ballabio A. The rapidly evolving view of lysosomal storage diseases. EMBO Mol Med. 2021;13:e12836.

46. Helmi MM, Saleh M, Yacop B, ElSawy D. Chédiak-Higashi syndrome with novel gene mutation. BMJ Case Reports. 2017;bcr2016216628.

47. Nagai K, Ochi F, Terui K, Maeda M, Ohga S, Kanegane H, et al. Clinical characteristics and outcomes of Chédiak-Higashi syndrome: A nationwide survey of Japan: Chédiak-Higashi Syndrome in Japan. Pediatr Blood Cancer. 2013;60:1582-6.

48. TchernevVT,MansfieldTA,GiotL,KumarAM,NandabalanK,LiY, et al. The Chediak-Higashi protein interacts with SNARE complex and signal transduction proteins. Mol Med. 2002;8:56-64.

49. Hollmann AK, Bleyer M, Tipold A, Neßler JN, Wemheuer WE, Schütz E, et al. A genome-wide association study reveals a locus for bilateraliridal hypopigmentation in Holstein Friesian cattle. BMC Genet. 2017;18:30.

50. Lin JY, Fisher DE. Melanocyte biology and skin pigmentation. Nature. 2007;445:843-50.

51. Tian X, Cui Z, Liu S, Zhou J, Cui R. Melanosome transport and regulationindevelopmentanddisease. PharmacolTher.2021;219:107707.

52. Tanabe F, Kasai H, Morimoto M, Oh S, Takada H, Hara T, et al. Novel heterogenous CHS1 mutations identified in five Japanese patients with Chediak-Higashi Syndrome. Case Rep Med. 2010;2010:464671.

53. Justiz Vaillant AA, Stang CM. Lymphoproliferative disorders. Treasure Island, FL: StatPearls Publishing; 2021.

54. Delplanque M, Galicier L, Oziol E, Ducharme-Bénard S,Oksenhendler E, Buob D, et al. AA amyloidosis secondary to primary immune deficiency: about 40 cases including 2 new French cases and a systematic literature review. J Allergy Clin Immunol Pract. 2021;9:745-52.

55. Fernández A, Hayashi M, Garrido G, Montero A, Guardia A, Suzuki T, et al. Genetics of non-syndromic and syndromic oculocutaneous albinisminhumanandmouse.PigmentCellMelanomaRes. 2021;34:786-99.

56. Kaplan J, De Domenico I, Ward DM. Chediak-Higashi syndrome. Curr Opin Hematol. 2008;15:22-9.

57. Thumbigere Math V, Rebouças P, Giovani PA, Puppin-Rontani RM, Casarin R, Martins L, et al. Periodontitis in Chédiak-Higashi Syndrome: an altered immunoinflammatory response. JDR Clin Trans Res. 2018;3:35- 46.

58. Weisfeld-Adams JD, Mehta L, Rucker JC, Dembitzer FR, Szporn A, Lublin FD, et al. Atypical Chédiak-Higashi syndrome with attenuated phenotype: three adult siblings homozygous for a novel LYST deletion and with neurodegenerative disease. Orphanet J Rare Dis. 2013;8:46.

59. Hedberg-Buenz A, Dutca LM, Larson DR, Meyer KJ, Soukup DA, van derHeide CJ, et al. Mouse models and strain-dependency of Chédiak- Higashi syndrome-associated neurologic dysfunction. Sci Rep. 2019;9:6752.

60. Buckley RM, Grahn RA, Gandolfi B, Herrick JR, Kittleson MD, BatemanHL,etal. Assistedreproductionmediresurrectionof afeline model for Chediak-Higashi syndrome caused by a large duplication in LYST. Sci Rep. 2020;10:64.

61. Gene Cards. LYST Gene - Lysosomal Trafficking Regulator. [Online]. 2021 [Accessed 05/01/2022], available at URL: https://www.genecards.org/cgi-bin/carddisp.pl?gene=LYST

62. Chan HW, Schiff ER, Tailor VK, Malka S, Neveu MM, Theodorou M, et al. Prospective study of the phenotypic and mutational spectrum of ocular albinism and oculocutaneous albinism. Genes (Basel). 2021;12:508.

63. Fukuchi K, Tatsuno K, Sakaguchi K, Sano S, Sasaki T, Aoki S, et al. Novel gene mutations in Chédiak-Higashi syndrome with hyperpigmentation. J Dermatol. 2019;46:e416-8.

64. Nagle DL, Karim MA, Woolf EA, Holmgren L, Bork P, Misumi DJ, et al. Identification and mutation analysis of the complete gene for Chediak-Higashi syndrome. Nat Genet. 1996;14:307-11.

65. Karim MA, Suzuki K, Fukai K, Oh J, Nagle DL, Moore KJ, et al. Apparent genotype-phenotype correlation in childhood, adolescent, and adult Chediak-Higashi syndrome. Am J Med Genet. 2002;108:16-22.

66. Barbosa M. Identification of mutations in two major mRNA isoforms of the Chediak- Higashi syndrome gene in human and mouse. Human Molecular Genetics. 1997;6:1091-8.

67. Karim MA, Nagle DL, Kandil HH, Bürger J, Moore KJ, Spritz RA. Mutations in the Chediak-Higashi syndrome gene (CHS1) indicate requirement for the complete 3801 amino acid CHS protein. Hum Mol Genet. 1997;6:1087-9.

68. Jessen B, Maul-Pavicic A, Ufheil H, Vraetz T, Enders A, Lehmberg K, et al. Subtle differences in CTL cytotoxicity determine susceptibility to hemophagocytic lymphohistiocytosis in mice and humans with Chediak-Higashi syndrome. Blood. 2011;118:4620-9.

69. Westbroek W, Adams D, Huizing M, Koshoffer A, Dorward H, Tinloy B, et al. Cellular defects in Chediak-Higashi syndrome correlate with the molecular genotype and clinical phenotype. J Invest Dermatol. 2007;127:2674-7.

70. Bhambhani V, Introne WJ, Lungu C, Cullinane A, Toro C. Chediak-Higashi syndrome presenting as young-onset levodopa-responsive parkinsonism: Parkinsonism in Chediak-Higashi Syndrome. Mov Disord. 2013;28:127-9.

71. Scherber E, Beutel K, Ganschow R, Schulz A, Janka G, Stadt U zur. Molecular analysis and clinical aspects of four patients with Chédiak- Higashi syndrome (CHS). Clin Genet. 2009;76:409-12.

72. Sánchez-Guiu I, Antón AI, García-Barberá N, Navarro-Fernández J, Martínez C, Fuster JL, et al. Chediak-Higashi syndrome: description of two novel homozygous missense mutations causing divergent clinical phenotype. Eur J Haematol. 2014;92:49-58.

73. Shimazaki H, Honda J, Naoi T, Namekawa M, Nakano I, Yazaki M, et al. Autosomal-recessive complicated spastic paraplegia with a novel lysosomal trafficking regulator gene mutation. J Neurol Neurosurg Psychiatry. 2014;85:1024-8.

74. Dufourcq-Lagelouse R, Lambert N, Duval M, Viot G, Vilmer E, Fischer A, et al. Chediak-Higashi syndrome associated with maternal uniparental isodisomy of chromosome 1. Eur J Hum Genet. 1999;7:633-7.

75. CertainS,BarratF,PasturalE,LeDeistF,Goyo-RivasJ,JabadoN,et al. Protein truncation test of LYST reveals heterogenous mutations in patients with Chediak-Higashi syndrome. Blood. 2000;95:979-83.

76. Manoli I, Golas G, WestbroekW, Vilboux T, Markello TC, Introne W, et al. Chediak-Higashi syndrome with early developmental delay resulting from paternal heterodisomy of chromosome 1. Am J Med Genet A. 2010;152A:1474-83.

77. Zarzour W, Kleta R, Frangoul H, Suwannarat P, Jeong A, Kim SY, et al. Two novel CHS1 (LYST) mutations: Clinical correlations in an infant with Chediak-Higashi syndrome. Mol Genet Metab. 2005;85:125-32.

78. Morrone K, Wang Y, Huizing M, Sutton E, White JG, Gahl WA, et al. Two novel mutations identified in an African-American child with Chediak-Higashi syndrome. Case Rep Med. 2010;2010:967535.

79. Barbosa MD, Nguyen QA, Tchernev VT, Ashley JA, Detter JC, Blaydes SM, et al. Identification of the homologous beige and Chediak- Higashi syndrome genes. Nature. 1996;382:262-5.

80. Al-Tamemi S, Al-Zadjali S, Al-Ghafri F, Dennison D. Chediak-Higashi syndrome: novel mutation of the CHS1/LYST gene in 3 Omani patients. J Pediatr Hematol Oncol. 2014;36:e248-50.

81. Gomaa NS, Lee JY, El Sharkawy A, El Chazli YF, Hassab HM, Doghaim NN, et al. Genetic analysis in Egyptian patients with Chediak-Higashi syndrome reveals new LYST mutations. Clin Exp Dermatol. 2019;44:814-7.

82. Aarts CE, Varga E, Webbers S, Geissler J, von Lindern M, Kuijpers TW, et al. Generation and characterization of a human iPSC lineSANi008- A from a Chédiak-Higashi Syndrome patient. Stem Cell Res. 2021;55:102442.

83. Faber IV, Prota JR, Martinez AR, Nucci A, Lopes-Cendes I, Júnior MC. Inflammatory demyelinating neuropathy heralding accelerated Chediak-Higashi syndrome. Muscle Nerve. 2017;55:756-60.

84. Arveiler B, Lasseaux E, Morice-Picard F. Clinicopathology and genetics of albinism. Presse Med. 2017;46:648-54.

85. Federico JR, Krishnamurthy K. Albinism. Treasure Island, FL: StatPearls Publishing; 2021.

86. Chin S, Kwon T, Khan BR, Sparks JA, Mallery EL, Szymanski DB, et al. Spatial and temporal localization of SPIRRIG and WAVE/SCAR reveal rolesforthese proteinsinactin-mediatedroothairdevelopment. PlantCell. 2021;33:2131-48.

87. Ridaura-Sanz C, Durán-McKinster C, Ruiz-Maldonado R. Usefulness of the skin biopsy as a tool in the diagnosis of silvery hair syndrome. Pediatr Dermatol. 2018;35:780-3.

88. Maaloul I, Talmoudi J, Chabchoub I, Ayadi L, Kamoun TH, Boudawara T, et al. Chediak-Higashi syndrome presenting in accelerated phase: A case report and literature review. Hematol Oncol Stem Cell Ther. 2016;9:71-5.

89. Zhang Y, Gao Z, Yu X. A case of Chediak-Higashi syndrome presented with accelerated phase could be treated effectively by unrelated cord blood transplantation. Pediatr Transplantation. 2017;21:e13014.

90. Dupuis A,BordetJC,Eckly A,GachetC. Platelet į-storagepool disease: an update. J Clin Med. 2020;9:2508.

91. Aarts CE, Downes K, Hoogendijk AJ, Sprenkeler EG, Gazendam RP, Favier R, et al. Neutrophil specific granule and NETosis defects in gray platelet syndrome. Blood Adv. 2021;5:549-64.

92. Nurden P, StrittS,FavierR, NurdenAT. Inheritedplatelet diseases with normal platelet count: phenotypes, genotypes and diagnostic strategy. Haematologica. 2021;106:337-50.

93. Yliranta A, Mäkinen J. Chediak-Higashi syndrome: neurocognitive and behavioral data from infancy to adulthood after bone marrow transplantation. Neurocase. 2021;27:1-7.

94. Shirazi TN, Snow J, Ham L, Raglan GB, Wiggs EA, Summers AC, et al. The neuropsychological phenotype of Chediak-Higashi disease. Orphanet J Rare Dis. 2019;14:101.

95. Koh K, Tsuchiya M,Ishiura H, Shimazaki H, Nakamura T, Hara H, et al. Chédiak-Higashi syndrome presenting as a hereditary spasticparaplegia. J Hum Genet. 2022;67:119-21.

96. Lolli V, Soto Ares G, Pruvo J-P, Abou Chahla W, Jissendi-Tchofo P. Chédiak-Higashi syndrome: brain MRI and MR spectroscopy manifestations. Pediatr Radiol. 2015;45:1253-7.

97. Gera A, Misra A, Tiwari A, Singh A, Mehndiratta S. A hungry histiocyte, altered immunity and myriad of problems: Diagnosticchallenges for pediatric HLH. Int J Lab Hematol. 2021;43:1443-50.

98. Lange M, Linden T, Müller HL, Flasskuehler MA, Koester H, Lehmberg K, et al. Primary haemophagocytic lymphohistiocytosis (Chédiak-Higashi Syndrome) triggered by acute SARS-CoV-2 infection in a six-week-old infant. Br J Haematol. 2021;195:198-200.

99. Soy M, Atagündüz P, Atagündüz I, Sucak GT. Hemophagocytic lymphohistiocytosis: a review inspired by the COVID-19 pandemic. Rheumatol Int. 2021;41:7-18.

100. CannaSW,MarshRA. Pediatrichemophagocyticlymphohistiocytosis. Blood.2020;135:1332-43.

101. Chinn IK, Eckstein OS, Peckham-Gregory EC, Goldberg BR, Forbes LR, Nicholas SK, et al. Genetic and mechanistic diversity in pediatric hemophagocytic lymphohistiocytosis. Blood. 2018;132:89-100.

102. Kim YR, Kim DY. Current status of the diagnosis and treatment of hemophagocytic lymphohistiocytosis in adults. Blood Res.2021;56(S1):17- 25.

103. Risma KA, Marsh RA. Hemophagocytic lymphohistiocytosis: clinical presentations and diagnosis. J Allergy Clin Immunol Pract. 2019;7:824-32.

104. Stolz W, GraubnerU, Gerstmeier J, Burg G, Belohradsky BH. Chdiak-Higashi Syndrome: Approaches in Diagnosis and Treatment. In: Fritsch P, Schuler G, Hintner H, eds. Current problems in dermatology. Basel: Karger; 1989.p.93-100.

105. SunY,LiY,HaoJ. Rareinclusionbodieswithinmonocytesataccelerated phaseofChediak-Higashisyndrome.ClinChemLabMed. 2018;56:e105-7.

106. Hoffmann J, Michel C, Schindler T, Wollmer E, Neubauer A. Seltene Erkrankungen am Blutbild erkennen. Internist (Berl). 2018;59:1106-13.

107. Kiyoi T, Liu S, Sahid MNA, Shudou M, Ogasawara M, Mogi M, et al. Morphological and functional analysis of beige (Chédiak-Higashi syndrome) mouse mast cells with giant granules. Int Immunopharmacol. 2019;69:202-12.

108. Zhang YH, Han X. Acute promyelocytic leukemia with Chediak-Higashi like giant granules. Blood. 2022;139:149.

109. Liu J, Dong SX, Li Y, Xu YD, Ru YX. Ultrastructural investigation on pseudo Chediak-Higashi abnormality in acute lymphoblastic leukemia: A case report. Pediatr Blood Cancer. 2021;69:e29541.

110. Zhong ZQ, Zhuang HF, Wu SL, Zhang H. Pseudo-Chédiak-Higashi inclusions in relapsed acute lymphoblastic leukaemia. Br J Haematol. 2021;195:300.

111. Kondo H, Kanayama T, Matsumura U, Urata T, Osone S, Imamura T, et al. Relapsed RUNX1-RUNX1T1-positive acute myeloid leukemia with pseudo-Chediak-Higashi granules. Int J Hematol. 2021;113:616-7.

112. Bouatay A, Hizem S, Tej A, Moatamri W, Boughamoura L, Kortas M. Chediak-higashi syndrome presented as accelerated phase: case report and review of the literature. Indian J Hematol Blood Transfus. 2014;30(Suppl 1):223-6.

113. Bhattarai D, Banday AZ, Sadanand R, Arora K, Kaur G, Sharma S, et al. Hair microscopy: an easy adjunct to diagnosis of systemic diseases in children. Appl Microsc. 2021;51:18.

114. Borges da Silva FA, Lorand-Metze I, Metze K. Chédiak-Higashi syndrome approached by several different microscopy imaging technologies. Br J Haematol. 2020;189:1001.

115. Griffin G, Shenoi S, Hughes GC. Hemophagocytic lymphohistiocytosis: An update on pathogenesis, diagnosis, and therapy. Best Pract Res Clin Rheumatol. 2020;34:101515.

116. Gopaal N, Sharma JN, Agrawal V, Lora SS, Jadoun LS. Chediak-Higashi syndrome with epstein-barr virus triggered hemophagocytic lymphohistiocytosis: a case report. Cureus. 2020;12:e11467.

117. Carter SJ, Tattersall RS, Ramanan AV. Macrophage activation syndrome in adults: recent advances in pathophysiology, diagnosis and treatment. Rheumatology (Oxford). 2019;58:5-17.

118. Kanjanapongkul S. Chediak-Higashi syndrome: report of a case with uncommon presentation and review literature. J Med Assoc Thai. 2006;89:541-4.

119. Nargund AR, Madhumathi DS, Premalatha CS, Rao CR, Appaji L, Lakshmidevi V. Accelerated phase of chediak higashi syndrome mimicking lymphoma - a case report. J Pediatr Hematol Oncol. 2010;32:e223-6.

120. Squire JD, Gardner PJ, Moutsopoulos NM, Leiding JW. Antibiotic Prophylaxis for Dental Treatment in Patients with Immunodeficiency. J Allergy Clin Immunol Pract. 2019;7:819-23.

121. Swaminathan VV, Uppuluri R, Meena SK, Varla H, Chandar R, Ramakrishnan B, et al. Treosulfan-based conditioning in matched family, unrelated and haploidentical hematopoietic stem cell transplantation for genetic hemophagocytic lymphohistiocytosis: experience and outcomes over10 yearsfromIndia.IndianJHematolBloodTransfus.2022;38:84-91.

122. GanesanN,KumarPN. Chediak-HigashiSyndromeinacceleratedphase. IndianJHematolBloodTransfus.2018;34:146-7.

123. Haddad E, Le DeistF, Blanche S, Benkerrou M, Rohrlich P, Vilmer E, et al. Treatment of Chediak-Higashi syndrome by allogenic bone marrow transplantation: report of 10 cases. Blood. 1995;85:3328-33.

124. Sachdev M, Bansal M, Chakraborty S, Hamal S, Bhargava R, Dua V. Haploidentical stem cell transplant with post-transplant cyclophosphamide for Chediak-Higashi Syndrome: a very rare case report. J Pediatr Hematol Oncol. 2021;43:e1030-2.

125. Dasouki M, Jabr A, AlDakheel G, Elbadaoui F, Alazami AM, Al‐Saud B, et al. TREC and KREC profiling as arepresentativeofthymus and bone marrowoutputin patients withvarious inbornerrors of immunity. Clin Exp Immunol. 2020;202:60-71.

126. Uppuluri R, Sivasankaran M, Patel S, Swaminathan VV, Ramanan KM, Ravichandran N, et al. Haploidentical stem cell transplantation with post-transplant cyclophosphamide for primary immune deficiencydisorders in children: challenges and outcome from a tertiary care center in South India. J Clin Immunol. 2019;39:182-7.

127. Shimizu K, Hayashi M, Ito N, Hamada K, Koizumi G, Kurohara K, et al. Oralmanagementofahaematopoieticstemcelltransplantrecipientwith Chédiak-Higashi Syndrome. Case Rep Dent. 2021;2021:9918199.

128. Bami S, Vagrecha A, Soberman D, Badawi M, Cannone D, Lipton JM, et al. The use of anakinra in the treatment of secondary hemophagocytic lymphohistiocytosis. Pediatr Blood Cancer. 2020;67:e28581.

129. Sadaat M, Jang S. Hemophagocytic lymphohistiocytosis with immunotherapy: brief review and case report. J Immunother Cancer. 2018;6:49.

130. La Rosée P, Horne A, Hines M, von Bahr Greenwood T, Machowicz R, Berliner N, et al. Recommendations for the management of hemophagocytic lymphohistiocytosis in adults. Blood. 2019;133:2465-77.

131. Créput C, Galicier L, Oksenhendler E, Azoulay E. Lymphohistiocytic activation syndrome: review of the literature, implications in intensive care. Reanimation. 2005;14:604-13.

132. Ehl S, Astigarraga I, von Bahr Greenwood T, Hines M, Horne A, Ishii E,etal. Recommendations fortheuseof etoposide-basedtherapyand bone marrowtransplantationforthetreatmentofHLH:ConsensusStatementsby the HLH Steering Committee of the Histiocyte Society. J Allergy Clin Immunol Pract. 2018;6:1508-17.

133. Zhuo W, Hao D, Tong Y, Wu W, Bao S, Huang K, et al. The occurrence and treatment of hemophagocytic lymphohistiocytosis caused by multiple factors: a case report and literature review. Ann Palliat Med.2021;10:3518- 23.

134. Keenan C, Nichols KE, Albeituni S. Use of the JAK inhibitor ruxolitinib in the treatment of hemophagocytic lymphohistiocytosis. Front Immunol. 2021;12:614704.

135. Jordan MB, Allen CE, Greenberg J, Henry M, Hermiston ML, Kumar A, et al. Challenges in the diagnosis of hemophagocytic lympho- histiocytosis: Recommendations from the North American Consortium for Histiocytosis (NACHO). Pediatr Blood Cancer. 2019;66:e27929.

136. Liu P, Pan X, Chen C, Niu T, Shuai X, Wang J, et al. Nivolumab treatment of relapsed/refractory Epstein-Barr virus-associated hemophagocytic lymphohistiocytosis in adults. Blood. 2020;135:826-33.

137. Mirza M, Zafar M, Nahas J, Arshad W, Abbas A, Tauseef A. Hemophagocytic lymph histiocytosis (HLH): etiologies, pathogenesis, treatment, and outcomes in critically ill patients: a review article and literature to review. J Community Hosp Intern Med Perspect. 2021;11:639- 45.

138. Cheloff AZ, Al-Samkari H. Emapalumab for the treatment of hemophagocyticlymphohistiocytosis.DrugsToday(Barc).2020;56:439-46.

139. Eloseily EM, Weiser P, Crayne CB, Haines H, Mannion ML, Stoll ML, et al. Benefit of anakinra in treating pediatric secondary hemophagocytic lymphohistiocytosis. Arthritis Rheumatol. 2020;72:326-34.

140. Astigarraga I, Gonzalez-Granado LI, Allende LM, Alsina L. Haemophagocytic syndromes: The importance of early diagnosis and treatment. An Pediatr (Engl Ed). 2018;89:124.e1-e8.

141. Vallurupalli M, Berliner N. Emapalumab for the treatment of relapsed/ refractory hemophagocytic lymphohistiocytosis. Blood. 2019;134:1783-6.

142. Bichon A, Bourenne J, Allardet-Servent J, Papazian L, Hraiech S, Guervilly C, et al. High mortality of HLH in ICU regardless etiology or treatment. Front Med (Lausanne). 2021;8:735796.

143. Tsuji T, Uemura Y, Nakamura Y, Nonoyama S. Oral mass revealing Chédiak-Higashi syndrome. Int J Oral Maxillofac Surg. 2017;46:1158-61.

144. Janka G, zur Stadt U. Familial and acquired hemophagocytic lympho-histiocytosis. Hematology Am Soc Hematol Educ Program. 2005:82-8.

145. Boussaadni YE, Benajiba N, Bousfiha AA, Ailal F. Macrophagic activation syndrome complicating familial lymphohistiocytosis. Pan Afr Med J. 2017;26:93.

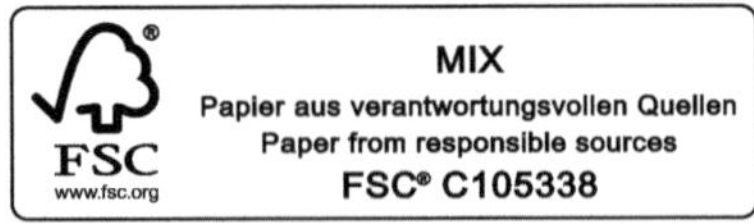

Printed by Books on Demand GmbH, Norderstedt / Germany